Intestinal Ischaemia

ERRATA

Marston—*Intestinal Ischaemia*

It is regretted that figures 2.2, 2.3, 6.1a and b and 6.5 have been printed upside down.

Intestinal Ischaemia

Adrian Marston

M.A., D.M., M.Ch., F.R.C.S.
Surgeon, The Middlesex and Royal Northern Hospitals,
London
Senior Lecturer in Surgery, University of London

With Illustrations by
Peter Drury, M.M.A.A.
Medical Illustrator, The Middlesex Hospital Medical
School, and Staff of the Department of Medical Illustration

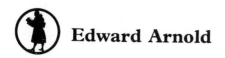
Edward Arnold

LAM J [Isve]

First published 1977
by Edward Arnold (Publishers) Ltd
25 Hill Street, London W1X 8LL

ISBN: 0 7131 4264 2

Printed in Great Britain by Butler & Tanner Ltd, Frome and London

Contents

Preface and Acknowledgement

This book is the outcome of a personal interest in the clinical and experimental aspects of intestinal ischaemia, which has extended over the last twenty years. It is designed to be a guide to the clinician and a route-map for the intending research worker, and represents, I hope, an outline of our present knowledge. It may seem presumptuous for one author to have attempted to cover this field, and in fact the task would have been quite impossible had I not made shameless use of my friends and colleagues. I have studied their patients, adopted their ideas, plagiarized their words and made extensive use of their illustrative material. I hope that I have not misinterpreted them, or anywhere failed to acknowledge my debt. The book is accordingly dedicated to my fellow authors:

Surgeons

John Bergan *Chicago*
Scott Boley *New York*
Gustav Bounous *Sherbrook*
David Cairns *London*
Robert Courbier *Marseille*
Lucien Deloyers *Brussels*
Harold Ellis *London*
Richard Gardham *Enfield*
Malcolm Gough *Oxford*
Mohamed Ahmed Hassan *Khartoum*
Leif Hulten *Göteborg*
Robert Kieny *Strasborg*
John Kinmonth *London*
Leslie Le Quesne *London*
Lyn Lockhart-Mummery *London*
Roger Marcuson *Manchester*
James Milliken *Dublin*
Francis Moore *Boston*
Robert Nevin *London*
Alan Parks *London*
George Parks *Belfast*
Cristobal Pera *Barcelona*
Murray Pheils *Sydney*
Colin Renton *Hereford*
Frédéric Saegesser *Lausanne*
Robert Shaw *Boston*

Douglas Short *Glasgow*
Kenneth Shute *London*
Henning Skjoldborg *Aarhus*
Michael Solan *Farnham*
Rafael Sobregrau *Barcelona*
Emeric Szilagyi *Detroit*
Gerald Taylor *London*
Richard Warren *Boston*
Lester Williams *Boston*
Colin Windsor *Worcester*

Physicians

Francis Avery-Jones *London*
Peter Ball *London*
Mario de Melos Bernado *Lisbon*
Jose Pinto Correia *Lisbon*
Elliot Corday *Los Angeles*
Peter Cotton *London*
Brian Creamer *London*
Anthony Dawson *London*
Jean-Pierre Delmont *Nice*
Peter Dick *Cambridge*
Donald Kellock *London*
Paul Kestens *Brussels*
Henri Sarles *Marseille*
Francisco Villardell *Barcelona*
John Vyden *Los Angeles*

Pathologists
Peter Antony   *London*
John Arthur   *Auckland*
Geoffrey Farrer-Brown   *London*
Richard Joske   *Perth*
Vincent McGovern   *Sydney*
Basil Morson   *London*
Charles Ross   *Chertsey*
Henry Thompson   *Birmingham*
Richard Whitehead   *Oxford*

Radiologists
Malcolm Chapman   *London*
Jack Farman   *New York*
Duncan Gregg   *Cambridge*
Hans Herlinger   *Leeds*
Michael Lea Thomas   *London*
Sol Schwartz   *New York*

Physiologists
Ove Lundgren   *Göteborg*
Eric Neil   *London*
Clinton Texter   *Little Rock*

My thanks are also due to my secretary, Yvonne Lim, who prepared the manuscript, to Mr R. R. Phillips and the Staff of the Department of Photography of The Middlesex Hospital, and to my younger son, Nicholas, who helped to compile the Index.

A.M.

I

Introduction

When medical scientists in different disciplines unexpectedly find themselves converging on the same area of study, the result is likely to be a profitable re-examination of previously accepted ideas. Such has been the case with ischaemic bowel disease as the result of three developments in medical thinking over the last thirty years.

1. Gastroenterologists suspected for some time that certain disorders of intestinal function were likely to be due to arterial insufficiency, much as happens in the heart, brain, kidney and other circulatory territories. Acute intestinal infarction resulting from mesenteric embolus and thrombosis had been recognized as a cause of death since the development of classical pathology in the mid-nineteenth century. It seemed likely that chronic obliterative disease of the visceral arteries could also occur and the existence of this disorder was speculated upon by such authors as Schnitzler[11] and Meyer.[10] However, as often happens, although a subject may have been extensively thought about and discussed in the literature, one observation suddenly illuminates the scene, and provides a starting point for scientific advance. In 1936 J. E. Dunphy, who was then a surgical resident at Peter Bent Brigham Hospital, published a paper[6] showing that the majority of patients dying of acute intestinal infarction gave a prodromal history of food-related abdominal colic, reminiscent of exercise pain felt in the ischaemic calf. From then on the concept of 'intestinal angina' had a respectable basis in pathology.

2. In the 1950s and early 60s the development of safe water-soluble contrast media and of retrograde arterial cannulation made it possible to map out the living arterial tree and to demonstrate sites of occlusion. The techniques of arterial suture and anastomosis, worked out years before by Carrel[3] in the experimental laboratory, then came into their own and began to be used on diseased human arteries with, at least in the short term, dramatic success. The first point of attack was the femoral artery, because this vessel is frequently occluded and is accessible to the surgeon. Moreover, the results of treatment are easy to assess because whether or not a patient claudicates, or whether or not a foot pulse is palpable, are recognized end-points which can be expressed in percentage terms of success or failure.

It soon became apparent, however, that to operate unselectively on every patient with claudication was mistaken, because in many cases the symptoms disappeared without treatment, and a failed operation could make the situation much worse, even to the extent of causing someone needlessly to lose a limb. The advent of new and enthusiastically applied surgical techniques provoked a critical re-examination of the natural history of the disease, and indeed it was argued by at least one school of thought[2] that arterial reconstruction had little if any part to play in the treatment of the ischaemic leg.

It was inevitable that, with new tools for diagnosis and treatment in their hands, surgeons sought to apply them to arteries other than those of the lower limb. The revelation that stroke was often related to lesions in the extracranial circulation, and hypertension to renal artery stenosis, led logically to an assault on the mesenteric circulation. However, the situation there was found to present certain difficulties. There was no clear-cut picture of the symptoms of arterial insufficiency in the gut. Abdominal pain is one of the most commonplace maladies of mankind, with a multitude of causes, many of which are emotionally rather than physically determined, and studies of post-mortem material[4] and of angiograms carried out for reasons other than suspected alimentary disease[5] showed that in fact the visceral arteries are very frequently the site of stenoses and occlusions which bear no discernible relationship to symptoms. Studies of intestinal function performed on patients with such occlusions usually fail to disclose any consistent derangement. In the laboratory animal also, it was shown that gradual obliteration of the blood supply to the gut was surprisingly well tolerated and could not be linked with any abnormality of structure or function, unless a fatal infarct was produced.[7]

Here, then, was an 'illness' with no clear-cut symptoms or physical signs, whose diagnosis depended on the radiographic demonstration of lesions which, it was admitted, were often symptomless, and whose treatment demanded a difficult and dangerous operation. It was scarcely surprising that sceptics poured scorn on the whole idea. However, the fact remained that acute midgut ischaemia was almost always fatal, and that as Dunphy had observed, and others confirmed, many of the victims gave a prodromal history which, if taken seriously, might have led to a timely preventive operation. What is more, each successive year brought a few reports showing how reconstructive arterial surgery could on occasion abolish abdominal pain and restore lost weight. The dilemma persists.

3. Over roughly the same period, pathologists were engaged in unravelling the tangled classification of inflammatory bowel disease. Apart from specific bacterial infections, two clear-cut 'granulomatous' syndromes were defined: ulcerative colitis (idiopathic proctocolitis) and Crohn's disease (regional enteritis). Although some overlap occurred, it appeared that these were two fundamentally different entities of separate causation, in each case quite undetermined. However, many cases of inflammatory bowel disease refused to fit into either category, and it seemed that some of these might in truth be of ischaemic origin. It was known from experimental studies[7, 8] that minor degrees of infarction could produce an acute inflammatory response in the bowel, but there appeared to be no clinical parallel. Such material was forthcoming in the late 1950s, when reports began to accumulate of the complications of aortic surgery[7] which showed that interference with the visceral arteries could lead to a spectrum of changes in the gut wall which were not only similar to those seen experi-

mentally, but also identical to hitherto unclassified types of inflammatory bowel disease. This led to the notion of 'ischaemic colitis' and 'ischaemic enterocolitis'[8] which are now universally accepted diagnostic categories.

However, the logical sequence of arterial blockage – ischaemia – bacterial invasion – inflammation – fibrosis cannot be the whole story, as in many cases of what may appear on clinical and pathological grounds to be ischaemic damage, no arterial occlusion can be found. It is commonplace to encounter lengths of gangrenous ileum and colon at an emergency operation, with vessels pulsating right up to the margin of the bowel. Similarly, selective angiography in the patient who presents the picture of ischaemic colitis may fail to reveal any arterial pathology, even when small vessels are catheterized and magnification techniques used.[1] This has led to the recognition of what has been termed 'non-occlusive' intestinal ischaemia. Why the intestine should on occasion undergo sudden necrosis in spite of a (grossly) normal blood supply is a mystery which has yet to be solved.

The chapters which follow are intended to bring together what is at present known of the ways in which the arterial supply to the alimentary tract can fail, and the clinical effects which result from such failure. There are several deliberate omissions, which have been made for the sake of uniformity. For instance, there are no separate chapters on radiology or histopathology, although it is of course true that without the help of these disciplines the whole subject of intestinal ischaemia would have remained unexplored. It none the less seemed better to include the radiographs and pathological illustrations along with the clinical and experimental material, seriatim. Also, the perinatal aspects of intestinal infarction are not discussed, nor are the possible relationships to blood flow of the colitis resulting from the newer antibiotics such as clindamycin and lincomycin. References are given, later in the text, to expert and specialized accounts of these aspects of the problem.

References

1 Baum, S. (1971). Normal anatomy and collateral pathways of the mesenteric circulation. In: *Vascular Disorders of the Intestine*, pp. 3–18. Ed. by S. J. Boley. New York and London, Appleton-Century-Crofts.
2 Bloor, K. (1961). Natural history of arteriosclerosis of the lower extremities. *Annals of the Royal College of Surgeons* **28**: 36–52.
3 Carrel, A. (1902). La technique opératoire des anastomoses vasculaires et la transplantations des viscères. *Lyon Medical* **98**: 859–870.
4 Derrick, J. R., Pollard, H. S. and Moore, R. M. (1959). The patterns of arteriosclerotic narrowing of the celiac and superior mesenteric arteries. *Annals of Surgery* **149**: 684–690.
5 Dick, A. P., Graffe, R., Gregg, D., Peter, N. and Sarner, M. (1967). An arteriographic study of mesenteric arterial disease: large vessel changes. *Gut* **8**: 206–211.
6 Dunphy, J. A. (1936). Abdominal pain of vascular origin. *American Journal of Medical Science* **192**: 109.

7   Marston, A. (1964). Patterns of intestinal ischaemia. *Annals of the Royal College of Surgeons* **35**: 151–157.

8   Marston, A., Pheils, M. T., Thomas, M. L. and Morson, B. C. (1966). Ischaemic colitis. *Gut* **7**: 1–10.

9   McGovern, V. J. and Goulstone, S. G. M. (1965). Ischaemic enterocolitis. *Gut* **6**: 213–220.

10   Meyer, J. (1924). Intermittent claudication (thromboangiitis obliterans) involving the intestinal tract. *Journal of the American Medical Association* **83**: 1414–1416.

11   Schnitzler, J. (1901). Zur Symptomalologie des damarterienverschlusses. *Münchener Medizinische Wochenschrift* **14**: 552.

12   Smith, R. F. and Szilagyi, D. E. (1960). Ischemia of the colon as a complication in the surgery of the abdominal aorta. *Archives of Surgery* **80**: 806–821.

2

Applied Anatomy of the Mesenteric Circulation

Introduction

This chapter is concerned with the gross and microscopic structure of the intestinal arteries, veins and lymphatics (lacteals), but mainly with the arteries, upon whose integrity depends the effective function of the alimentary tract as an absorptive, excretory, propulsive and endocrine organ. The basic outlines of this complicated structure were worked out by the classical anatomical studies of over a hundred years ago[21] using the Vesalian techniques of formal cadaveric dissection. However, the static architecture revealed by such methods tells us little about the working of the living, moving human body, and nothing of the subvisual components of the circulation on which function depends. To conventional dissections have now been added radiological studies,[4, 22, 25] using selective arterial catheterization, and examination of the microcirculation, by means of corrosion casts and injections of particles of known diameter.

There are three components to the splanchnic arterial tree. First are the *main vessels* arising from the aorta, which are of great clinical importance but, because pressure within them is virtually identical to central (left ventricular) pressure, have little influence on blood flow.[11] Second are the visible, surgically accessible, vessels, on which segmental blood flow depends, knowledge of whose anatomy is essential in clinical practice – referred to in this book as the *intermediate vessels*. The *microcirculation* is the final common pathway of arteries, capillaries and venules, and has a lymphatic component. Events here, the actual territory of oxygen exchange, are the true determinants of intestinal function.[26]

The main arteries

The three main visceral arteries correspond to the embryological areas of the gastrointestinal tract: the foregut, midgut and hindgut. Of these, much the largest is the midgut, which is that part of the alimentary tract which emerges into the yolk sac during the eighth week of fetal life, on the axis of its main vessel, the superior mesenteric artery (SMA) (Fig. 2.1). The arteries to the foregut (the coeliac axis) and the hindgut (the inferior mesenteric artery) convey relatively less blood to the intestine, and, through collateral pathways, their distribution extends over into extra-coelomic structures (Fig. 2.2). Patterns of blood supply to the gut are very variable, and in only 50 per cent of cases is the 'classical' arrangement found.[5] For this reason it is sometimes difficult to distinguish between

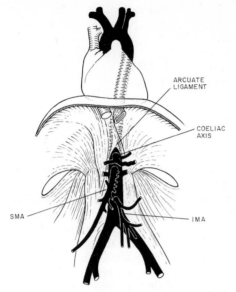

Fig. 2.1. Diagram of the main visceral arteries.

what is an anatomical variant and what is an abnormality caused by disease.[4, 24, 26]

The coeliac axis

The coeliac axis is a short, stumpy tube which runs straight out of the front of the aorta at the level of the first lumbar vertebra. Its origin is crossed by the fibres of the arcuate ligament of the diaphragm, and by a network of sympathetic nerves, the coeliac ('solar') plexus. The vessel may be kinked at this point, and show a post-stenotic dilatation below. The clinical significance of this variant has caused dispute.

Almost immediately, the axis divides into its three branches.

The splenic artery

This runs upwards and to the left along the upper border of the body and tail of the pancreas, and then enters the hilum of the spleen where it divides into four to twelve branches, some of which supply the spleen substance and others run as the vasa brevia to the greater curve of the stomach, where they anastomose with the left gastroepiploic artery. The splenic artery is unusual in that it does not run a direct straight course but is wavy and tortuous throughout its length. This feature can sometimes be put to surgical use, in that the spleen may be removed and the splenic artery mobilized, straightened out and brought down to other parts of the mesenteric circulation to irrigate an ischaemic area.

The left gastric artery

This runs directly forwards from the coeliac axis to reach the midpoint of the lesser curve of the stomach. Here it divides into upper and lower branches. The upper branch supplies the upper part of the lesser curve, and anastomoses with the phrenic branches of the aorta, the lower intercostals and the oesophageal arteries. The lower branch runs down to anastomose with the right gastric artery in the region of the pyloric antrum. This artery sometimes gives important supply to the liver via a left hepatic artery running across the lesser omentum.

The hepatic artery

This runs to the right, along the upper border of the head of the pancreas, to the first part of the duodenum. Here it gives off the large and important *gastroduodenal artery*, which grooves the pancreas as it runs down behind the first part of the duodenum to supply that structure and the head and uncinate process of the pancreas. The main trunk of the hepatic artery turns upwards and to the right to enter the free edge of the lesser omentum, in a variable relationship to the portal vein and common bile duct, but usually anteriorly and to the left. It passes up to the hilum of the liver and divides into right and left branches which supply the respective 'lobes' of the liver which do not, however, always correspond with the pattern of venous and biliary drainage.

In the non-cirrhotic liver some two-thirds of the oxygen and nutritional requirements are met by the portal vein, so that occlusion of the hepatic artery is relatively well tolerated. It used to be thought that interruption of this vessel led inevitably to necrosis of the liver, but such is not in fact

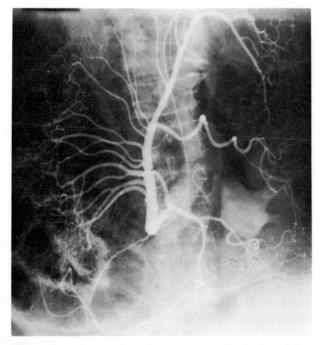

Fig. 2.2. Selective angiogram showing normal distribution of the superior mesenteric artery (by courtesy of Dr Hans Herlinger).

the case, and the hepatic artery is quite frequently tied deliberately, as part of the treatment of metastatic tumours. Conversely, when the SMA is occluded, the hepatic artery may contribute significantly to the blood supply of the gut, without any deleterious effect on liver function.

The superior mesenteric artery

The SMA is the crucial and all-important vessel of the alimentary tract. It arises from the front of the aorta, usually just above the renal arteries and at the level of the L1/2 intervertebral disc. At its origin it is 1–1·5 cm in diameter. It runs immediately in front of the neck of the pancreas, crosses behind the uncinate process, and then passes in front of the third part of the duodenum to enter the mesentery of the small intestine. This area can sometimes be seen on a barium study as a band of translucency running vertically across the duodenum. If the proximal duodenum appears at all dilated, this normal finding may be misinterpreted as representing an obstruction, to which clinical symptoms are then attributed. In fact the syndrome of 'duodenal ileus' has little factual evidence to sustain it, and has never been confirmed by endoscopy. This band of translucency probably also accounts for the mythical 'sphincter of Ochsner' analogous to the high pressure zones at the ileocaecal valve and the rectosigmoid junction. There is, however, some evidence that pressure defects on the duodenal loop are of significance when the SMA is occluded.[1]

Just as the left hepatic artery can arise from the left gastric, so the *right hepatic artery* may originate as the first branch of the superior mesenteric, running up under the uncinate process and through the pancreas.[27]

The first branch of the SMA is the *inferior pancreatoduodenal artery*, which passes up behind the head of the pancreas to join the *superior pancreatoduodenal branch* of the gastroduodenal artery. These small vessels have considerable clinical importance. In the first place, they provide a major part of the blood supply to the head of the pancreas and the lower part of the common bile duct, and thus must be carefully preserved whenever the pancreas is partially resected. More important, this anastomosis represents the main collateral pathway between the arterial territories of the coeliac axis and the superior mesenteric artery, and is capable of a remarkable degree of dilatation if the SMA becomes occluded (see Figs. 2.12 and 2.13).

The origin of the SMA, lying well back in the upper part of the abdominal cavity and surrounded by pancreas, sympathetic nerve fibres, portal vein and duodenum, is one of the most inaccessible structures in the human body. It is almost impossible to expose it without a full thoracoabdominal incision, which constitutes a very major anatomical insult. For this reason, operations on this area are best avoided, and wherever possible the vascular problem is solved by an indirect approach.

Emerging from behind the duodenum, the SMA passes downwards in the root of the small bowel mesentery towards the right iliac fossa, usually with a left-sided convexity. The first branch after the inferior pancreatoduodenal artery is the *middle colic artery*, which springs from the right side of the vessel, enters the transverse mesocolon and divides into left and right branches which constitute part of the important marginal supply to the colon (see below). *The right colic artery*, which is usually quite small, arises some 4 cm further down, and the *ileocolic* some 4 cm below that. The main trunk of the SMA passes downwards to enter the marginal colonic circulation in the ileocaecal region, and anastomoses with the terminal branches of the ileocolic artery. Of these three right-sided colonic vessels, the only constant artery is the ileocolic,[27] which supplies the base of the right colon via anterior and posterior caecal arteries, terminal ileal branches and the small but clinically vital appendicular artery. The right and middle colic arteries have a variable pattern of origin from the main trunk[27] and often arise in common. In 10 per cent of cases the right colic artery arises from the ileocolic.

The small bowel circulation comes from the left side of the SMA via the so-called 'intestinal arteries' which vary in number between three and twenty, and from a series of arcades which increase in number and complexity from above downwards (see Fig. 2.4).

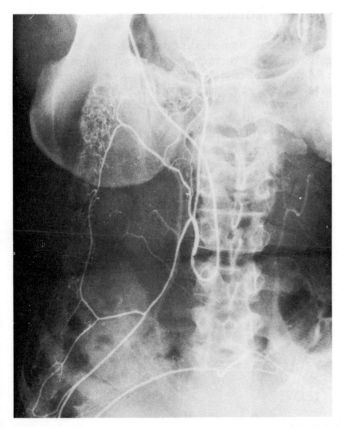

Fig. 2.3. Selective angiogram showing normal distribution of the inferior mesenteric artery (by courtesy of Dr Hans Herlinger).

The inferior mesenteric artery

The inferior mesenteric artery (IMA) (Fig. 2.3) is a very much smaller vessel than is the coeliac axis or SMA. It arises from the left anterior face of the aorta some 4 cm above the bifurcation, and for the first 2 cm of its course is usually buried within the aortic wall. Typically, it then gives off one or two downward-running branches to the sigmoid colon, and an important upward-running left colic artery, which gives rise to three to four *vasa recta* before joining the marginal artery to the colon. It then runs downwards behind the recto-sigmoid junction and rectum, and ends as the *superior haemorrhoidal artery* which divides into three major arterial trunks, one on the left and two on the right. The collateral circulation from the branches of the internal iliac artery (that is to say, the middle haemorrhoidal branch of the pudendal artery) anastomose very freely with this lower territory of the inferior mesenteric.

The intermediate arteries

Lying between the major aortic branches and the microscopic vessels and plexuses supplying the intimate structures, there is a network of anatomically visible trunks which are of clinical importance because they may be the seat of intrinsic disease or may be damaged by incidental or surgical trauma. This intermediate circulation comprises the intestinal vessels and the arcade systems of the small bowel, and the marginal circulation and the vasa recta of the colon. Interruption of an individual vessel in this system produces no damage to the mucosal circulation nor to the function of the bowel. However, if several vessels are involved, as may occur from embolus or atheromatous thrombosis, from a wound of the mesentery or

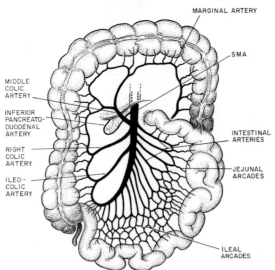

Fig. 2.4. Diagram of the intermediate vessels to the small bowel.

a badly planned surgical resection, or from an intramesenteric haematoma, there may result very considerable damage to the intestine, to the extent of actual necrosis (see Chapter 7).

The pattern of distribution of the intermediate vessels to the small bowel is represented in Fig. 2.4. The intermediate vessels to the large bowel are, however, of greater clinical importance.

The marginal artery to the colon

This is formed by the union of the three main colonic branches, which arise from the right side of the SMA, and which then continue around the splenic flexure to join the upward-running left colic branch of the IMA. This is a very important vessel, whose detailed anatomy has been accurately worked out only comparatively recently.[3, 20, 25, 27]

The arrangement of vessels along the right colon is fairly constant, there being one marginal artery giving off vasa recta and vasa brevia which occasionally communicate, though the anastomoses are much less developed than in the arcades of the small bowel. It is at the point of junction of superior and inferior mesenteric systems (at the splenic flexure) that confusion and variability occur.

The IMA divides into two or three branches, the uppermost of which (left colic) almost always reaches the splenic flexure. Here it bifurcates, the slender outer branch joining the left branch of the middle colic to form the marginal artery (of Drummond) of the colon, the inner (larger) branch running back into the trunk of the middle colic artery to form an additional arcade, the arc of Riolan (Fig. 2.5). The outer anastomosis is here often very small or incomplete, so that the continuity of the marginal artery is broken. If the arc of Riolan is not well developed, there exists here a critical area of anastomotic supply, so that impairment of flow in either SMA or

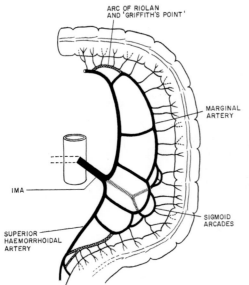

Fig. 2.5. Diagram of the intermediate vessels to the large bowel.

IMA will not be compensated, and may result in ischaemic damage. This is borne out by the frequency of ischaemic lesions at the splenic flexure (see below).

Where there is a requirement for collateral flow, the arc of Riolan will dilate according to a number of well established radiological patterns[29, 32] (see below). There are also a number of aberrant arteries which supply this area of the colon, arising as primary anatomical variations or from alterations in pressure and flow resulting from occlusions. These have been well summarized by Michels[27] and include a common coeliacomesenteric trunk, a splenocolic trunk whereby the middle colic artery comes off the splenic, and a common hepatocolic trunk. Bearing in mind the very complex train of embryological events which determine the final pattern of blood supply to an organ, it is hardly surprising that variants should exist, and the exact percentage incidence of the different arrangements encountered is of more academic than clinical interest.

The rectal blood supply is furnished by the lower branches of the IMA, supplemented by the contributions of the internal iliac artery via its middle and inferior haemorrhoidal branches (Fig. 2.6). The sigmoidal branches of the IMA number from one to five, depending on the length of this loop of colon. The extent of anastomosis between the individual branches is

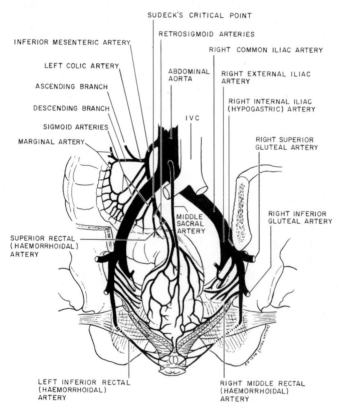

Fig. 2.6. Diagram of the intermediate vessels in the pelvis.

variable, but is less important than higher up in the bowel because of the rich communication with the internal iliac system. It used to be taught that a critical point[37] existed between the last sigmoid branch and the superior haemorrhoidal arteries, but more detailed anatomical studies by Griffiths[20] and others[3, 4, 6, 29, 32] have shown that this is not the case.

The terminal vessels to the hindgut are the *middle* and *inferior rectal arteries*.

The middle rectal artery arises either directly from the internal iliac or from one of its main divisions, and usually anastomoses with the lower branches of the IMA outside the rectal wall.

The inferior rectal artery arises constantly from the inferior pudendal, below the origin of the levator ani muscle, and supplies blood to the lower, non-endodermal parts of the alimentary tract, that is to say the anal canal with its intrinsic and extrinsic muscles, and the ischiorectal fossa. It anastomoses freely with the superior and middle rectal arteries and also with the median sacral artery (vestigial in man, but of great importance in caudate animals).

As in the small bowel, the colonic arcade gives rise to *vasa recta* which pass around alternate aspects of the colon, then divide into anterior and posterior branches which run to the edges of the antimesenteric taeniae, where they again divide, and pierce the circular muscle. From the origins of the vasa recta the *vasa brevia* run to the mesenteric attachment, anastomose there, and finally pierce the muscle on either side of the mesenteric taenia[6] (Fig. 2.7).

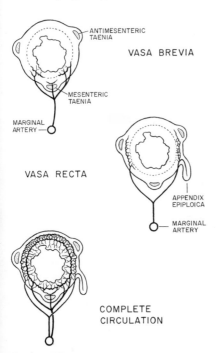

Fig. 2.7. The vasa recta and the vasa Brevia.

The microcirculation

The intramural vessels

Small branches arise from both vasa recta and vasa brevia to supply the peritoneum, and the appendices epiploicae. Additionally, a plexus (the external muscular plexus) is formed just beneath the serosa.

Having pierced the muscle, the arteries form a rich submucosal plexus, from which a few recurrent branches run back into the muscle,[7, 34] and may join the external muscular plexus.

The submucosal plexus extends as a continuous network over the length

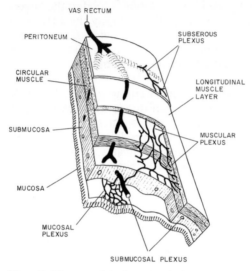

Fig. 2.8. Diagram of the intramural plexuses.

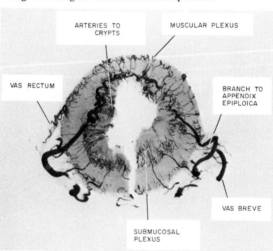

Fig. 2.9. Injected specimen showing the intramural plexuses of the colon.

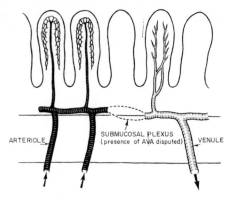

Fig. 2.10. The minute vessels.

of the bowel, and is composed of a coarse meshwork arranged in roughly rectangular pattern. Between the vessels in this network there lies a smaller, finer mesh from which spring the arterioles running up the villi, or between the crypts, to supply the mucous membrane itself. The submucosal plexus is richer and better developed in the small intestine than in the colon,[16, 34] which helps to explain the former's capacity to withstand ischaemic insult.[16, 17] In addition, some authors distinguish a distinct 'mucosal plexus' lying beneath the muscularis mucosae of the small bowel.[7, 31]

Arteriovenous anastomoses
The significance of arteriovenous anastomoses (AVA) is disputed. Although Spanner[33] was confident of his demonstration of arteriovenous connections in the submucous plexus of the gut wall, modern authorities are less certain.[8, 9] Such anastomoses are not easy to identify, and injection techniques may give misleading results.[35] Most authors seem to agree that they are few and far between, and probably not of great functional importance. These communications are more easily demonstrated in the stomach and colon than in the small bowel,[1, 2, 8, 9] though their existence even here has been disputed.[13]

The circulation to the villus

Vessels from the submucosal plexus contribute a single arteriole to each villus, about 20 μm in diameter, which runs up the central stroma and becomes capillarized (in other words, loses its smooth muscle coat) at a short distance beyond its base. As the tip of the villus is approached, the arteriole begins to arborize, and eventually divides into a very complicated system of fine subepithelial channels, which eventually drain into a central vein.

The relationship between the minute arteries and minute veins in the villous circulation is extremely close, and how much actual anatomical shunting takes place has for long been a matter of debate. This is of crucial importance in the maintenance of the mucosal circulation in hypotensive states, and in the production of pseudomembranes, as is discussed below.

The arterial and venous loops in the villi are arranged in much the same 'hairpin' pattern as is seen in the nephron. An additional factor is the presence of a central lymphatic, which carries a considerable volume of fluid, and has an effect, as yet undetermined, on total tissue flow. There is evidence of a countercurrent exchange of oxygen and nutrients in the intestinal villus much as happens with solutes in the nephron. Also, Horstmann[23] has shown that the aspect of the capillary which faces the epithelium is thin and contains pores, whereas the opposite side is thicker, without pores, and bears the cell nucleus.

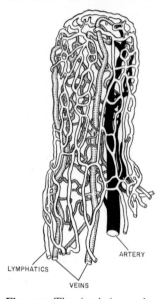

ARTERY

LYMPHATICS

VEINS

Fig. 2.11. The circulation to the villus (by courtesy of Dr O. Lundgren).

Pathological anatomy and collateral pathways

The coeliac axis

The coeliac axis may be occluded by atheroma, fibromuscular hyperplasia, or by a malignant tumour,[12] but the usual anatomical lesion is compression by the fibres of the arcuate ligament of the diaphragm, which may or may not give rise to symptoms.[18] The distal branches of the coeliac axis are rarely affected by arterial disease.

The territory irrigated by the coeliac axis[38] has a rich collateral supply from:

1. The lower intercostal branches, via the abdominal wall.
2. The phrenic branches of the aorta.

3. The lower oesophageal arteries, which perfuse the fundus and upper part of the body of the stomach, via the mucosal and submucosal plexuses.
4. The SMA, via the pancreatic arcades (see below).

From this it follows that occlusion of the axis, provided it does not occur too abruptly and that the SMA is intact, results in comparatively little disturbance in blood flow to the upper abdominal organs. The few flow studies which have been carried out in cases of coelic axis compression do not suggest any major degree of ischaemia, such as would interfere with function.[19]

The superior mesenteric artery

The SMA is either totally or partially occluded in two-thirds of people over the age of 55, as determined by random autopsy and radiological studies.[10, 15] Furthermore, because of its angle of emergence from the aorta, it accepts emboli with readiness, and mesenteric embolus has been a classically recognized complication of atrial fibrillation, mural thrombosis of the left ventricle, and aortic atheroma.

In contrast to what obtains in the coeliac axis, the upper and lower routes of collateral supply to the main midgut loop are ill developed and precarious. If the main trunk is occluded, the midgut is perfused from above via the mucosal plexuses of the duodenum, which are supplied in turn partly by the gastric and gastroepiploic arcades, and partly from extracoelomic vessels. The most obvious route of supply is via the pancreatic arcades, which can hypertrophy to a very striking degree (Figs. 2.12, 2.13). There may be a single or a double connecting channel between SMA and coeliac axis, depending on the configuration of the superior and inferior pancreatoduodenal arteries.[27, 29] Less conspicuously, the dorsal pancreatic artery,[29] which may originate from either SMA or coeliac axis, can carry blood backwards if either main trunk is blocked.

These routes of perfusion, when combined, may allow as much as

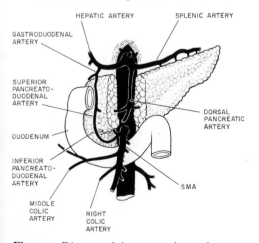

Fig. 2.12. Diagram of the pancreatic arcade system.

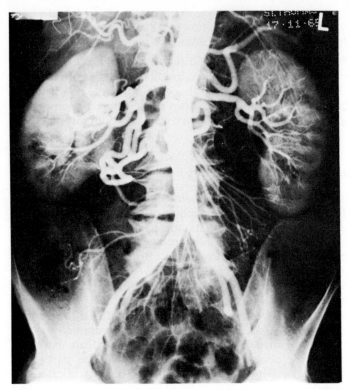

Fig. 2.13. Angiogram showing dilatation of the pancreatic arcade following obstruction of the SMA.

25–30 cm of jejunum to remain viable when the superior mesenteric artery has been abruptly occluded. Indeed, it is rare for the whole of the upper midgut loop to undergo necrosis following a mesenteric embolus. When the blockage occurs more gradually, development of other anastomotic channels may support a small intestine which shows no structural abnormality whatever (see Chapter 6).

From below, the contribution of the SMA is augmented by blood arriving from the marginal and intramural circulations of the colon. The main route of supply here is, of course, the inferior mesenteric artery,[28] via the anastomotic circulation already described, but the large intestine also obtains a variable quantity of arterial blood from the abdominal wall. Occlusion of the SMA, therefore, affects the colon when (1) the block has occurred proximal to the origin of the middle colic artery, or (2) the IMA is occluded.

The inferior mesenteric artery

The IMA although often atherosclerotic,[14] is, for practical purposes, never the site of an embolus. Occlusion close to its origin is well tolerated. The main surgical importance of the IMA is its involvement in atheromatous abdominal aneurysms, and the correct site of its ligation in the course of colonic resections.

The vessel is almost always interrupted during the repair of an abdominal aortic aneurysm, as it arises from the sac. The artery will often have been already blocked but, even if it is still patent, it can usually be safely tied, provided that the ligature is applied in the intra-aortic part of the vessel. This preserves the vital sigmoid branches and the marginal circulation to the colon. Nevertheless, there is a certain incidence of ischaemic damage to the large bowel following aortic reconstruction, which will be discussed below (see Chapter 6), and some surgeons recommend that the IMA should be reimplanted into the prosthesis.

The very rich route of collateral supply to the anal canal and lower rectum via the internal iliac arteries has already been described.

Comparative anatomy of the mesenteric circulation

This was investigated by Noer.[30] He showed that, whereas the SMA is the sole route of supply to the midgut loop in all mammals, there are considerable species differences where the distal circulation is concerned. On the whole the chimpanzee, the opossum and, to a lesser extent, the rabbit resemble man, but the dog, cat and other carnivores are quite different. Nevertheless, almost all experimental work in this field has been carried out on dogs and cats.

There seems surprisingly little correlation, however, between arterial pattern and food habits.

The main differences between dog and man are these:

1. The dog has a common colic artery which arises above the inferior pancreatoduodenal and supplies the whole colon.
2. The vasa recta intercommunicate in the dog.
3. The number of arcades in the dog remain few and fairly constant from jejunum to ileum.
4. The subserosal plexus is much less well developed.

The veins and lymphatics

The anatomy of the effluent vessels of the intestinal tract has received little study, as they follow so closely the paths of the arteries. The alimentary veins are notable in that they contain no valves, so that flow can take place in either direction and changes in portal pressure are communicated directly to the gut wall. In other words, tissue pressure in the intestine is influenced by events in the liver rather than in the systemic circulation. The portal system of veins is of large capacity and in many species can expand and 'pool' a considerable proportion of the blood volume. This probably does not take place in man.

The lymphatics here have a special role to play in that, rather than simply draining tissue fluid, they are a major route of absorption of nutrients. The osmotic effect of chyle is much greater than that of lymph, and exerts a large (though hitherto unmeasured) effect on the exchange of substances within the villus. The mesenteric lymphatics converge into the major lymph trunks on the posterior abdominal wall and eventually, via the cisterna chyli and the thoracic duct, deliver their contents into the venous system at the root of the neck.

References

1   Barclay, A. and Bentley, S. H. (1949). The vascularisation of the human sto-mach. *British Journal of Radiology* **22**: 62–67.
2   Barlow, T. E. (1951). Arteriovenous anastomoses in the human stomach. *Journal of Anatomy* **85**: 1–5.
3   Basmajian, J. V. (1954). The marginal anastomosis of the arteries to the large intestine. *Surgery, Gynecology and Obstetrics* **99**: 614–616.
4   Baum, S., Stein, G. N. and Baue, A. (1965). Extrinsic pressure defects on the duodenal loop in mesenteric occlusive disease. *Radiology* **85**: 866–871.
5   Baum, S. (1971). Normal anatomy and collateral pathways of the mesenteric circulation. In: *Vascular Disorders of the Intestine*, pp. 3–18. Ed. by S. J. Boley. New York and London, Appleton-Century-Crofts.
6   Benjamin, H. B. and Becker, A. B. (1959). A vascular study of the small in-testine. *Surgery, Gynecology and Obstetrics* **108**: 134–140.
7   Bernardo, M. O. de M. (1974). Alguns aspectos da vascularizacao parietal do colon. *Thesis*, University of Lisbon, pp. 46–47.
8   Boulter, P. S. and Parks, A. G. (1960). Submucosal vascular patterns of the alimentary tract and their significance. *British Journal of Surgery* **47**: 546–549.
9   Brockis, J. G. and Moffat, D. B. (1958). The intrinsic blood vessels of the pelvic colon. *Journal of Anatomy* **92**: 52–56.
10 Carucci, J. J. (1953). Mesenteric vascular occlusion. *American Journal of Surgery* **85**: 47–51.
11 Caudwell, E. W. and Anson, B. J. (1943). Visceral branches of the abdominal aorta. *American Journal of Anatomy* **73**: 27–34.
12 Cornell, S. H. Severe stenosis of the coeliac axis. *Radiology* **99**: 311–313.
13 Delaney, J. P. (1975). The paucity of arteriovenous anastomoses in the stomach. *Surgery* **78**: 411–413.
14 Demos, N. J., Bahuth, J. J. and Urnes, P. D. (1962). Comparative study of arteriosclerosis in the inferior and superior mesenteric arteries. *Annals of Surgery* **155**: 599–606.
15 Derrick, J. R., Pollard, H. S. and Moore, R. M. (1959). The patterns of arterio-sclerotic narrowing of the celiac and superior mesenteric arteries. *Annals of Surgery* **149**: 684–689.
16 Donnellan, W. L. (1965). The structure of the colonic mucosa. *Gastroenterology* **49**: 496–501.
17 Doran, F. S. A. (1950). Intramural blood supply of upper jejunum in man. *Journal of Anatomy* **84**: 283–286.
18 Dunbar, J. D. (1965). Compression of the coeliac trunk and abdominal angina. *American Journal of Roentgenology* **95**: 731–735.
19 Edwards, A. J. and Taylor, G. W. (1970). Experience with the coeliac axis com-pression syndrome. *British Medical Journal* **1**: 1342–1345.
20 Griffiths, J. D. (1961). Extramural and intramural blood supply of the colon. *British Medical Journal* **1**: 323–326.
21 Heller, A. (1872). Uber de Blutgefasse des Dunndarmes. *Berliner Sachsiger gesamte Wissenschaft* **24**: 165–171.

22 Herlinger, H. (1972). Angiography of the visceral arteries. *Clinics in Gastroenterology* **1**: 547–579.
23 Horstmann, E. (1966). Uber das Endothel der Zothenkapillaren im Dünndarm des Meerschweinchen und des Menschen. *Zeitschrift für Zellforschung* **72**: 364–369.
24 Imperati, L. and Tommaseo, T. (1960). *Chirurgia delle Arterie Mesenteriche.* Rome, Edizioni Mediche & Scientifiche.
25 Kahn, P. and Abrams, H. L. (1964). Inferior mesenteric arterial patterns—an angiographic study. *Radiology* **82**: 429–441.
26 Marston, A. (1972). Basic structure and function of the intestinal circulation. *Clinics in Gastroenterology* **1**: 439–546.
27 Michels, N. A. (1955). *Blood Supply and Anatomy of Upper Abdominal Organs with Descriptive Atlas.* Philadelphia, Pa., J. B. Lippincott Co.
28 Moskowitz, M., Zimmerman, H. and Felson, B. (1964). The meandering mesenteric artery of the colon. *American Journal of Roentgenology* **92**: 1088–1099.
29 Nebesar, R. A., Kornblith, P. L., Pollard, J. J. and Michels, N. A. (1969). *Celiac and Superior Mesenteric Arteries: a correlation of angiograms and dissections.* Boston, Mass., Little Brown & Co.
30 Noer, R. J. (1943). The blood vessels of the jejunum and ileum—a comparative study of man and certain laboratory animals. *American Journal of Anatomy* **73**: 3–293.
31 Patzelt, V. (1936). *Handbuch der Mikroscopischen Anatomie des Menschens*, pp. 1–448. Ed. W. V. Mollendorf. Berlin, Springer Verlag.
32 Reiner, L., Jimenez, F. A. and Rodriguez, F. L. (1963). Atherosclerosis in the mesenteric circulation. *American Heart Journal* **66**: 200–209.
33 Spanner, R. Neue Befunde über die Blutwege der Darmwand und ihre funktionelle Bedeutung. *Morphologische Jahrbuch* **69**: 394–454.
34 Spjut, H. J., Margulis, A. R. and McAlister, W. H. (1964). Microangiographic study of gastrointestinal lesions. *American Journal of Roentgenology* **92**: 1173–1187.
35 Staubesand, J. and Hammersen, F. (1956). Zur Problematik des Nachweises Arterio-Venöser Anastomosen im Injektionspräparat. *Zeitschrift für die gesamte Anatomie* **119**: 365–370.
36 Steward, J. A. and Rankin, F. W. (1933). Blood supply of large intestine: its surgical considerations. *Archives of Surgery* **26**: 843.
37 Sudeck, P. (1907). Uber die Gefässversorgung des Mastdarmes im Hinsicht auf die Operative Gangrän. *München medizinische Wochenschrift* **54**: 13–14.
38 Tandler, J. (1904). Uber die Varietäten der Arteria Coelica und deren Entwickelung. *Anatomische Hefte* **25**: 472–477.

3

Regulation and Distribution of Intestinal Blood Flow

Introduction

The circulatory volume is conventionally divided into six components, which supply blood to the brain, heart, kidneys, skeletal muscles, skin and abdominal organs. The last of these (the splanchnic circulation) is anatomically defined by the arteries and veins which have been described in the preceding chapter, and is subdivided into hepatic, splenic, and mesenteric circulations, which subserve different functions and do not always act in unison. The volume of blood which any one such compartment or subcompartment obtains will depend on the over-all blood volume, the cardiac output, the arterial pressure and other centrally determined factors, but the share which is devoted to a particular region is a function of locally regulated vascular resistances. Studies of the mesenteric circulation therefore need to take into account the blood volume, the cardiac output, the proportion of that output reaching the alimentary tract per unit time (i.e. the blood flow), the way in which the flow may change, and the manner in which it is distributed between the various layers of the gut.

The design of the intestinal circulation has to cope with environmental extremes. On the one hand is the active, running animal pursuing or being pursued, whose survival depends on adequate nutrition of its central nervous system and skeletal muscle, and whose skin and gut can for the moment safely be deprived of blood. In contrast, the resting beast, concerned with digesting and absorbing its fodder or prey, requires an alimentary tract full of arterial blood to ensure efficient propulsion and absorption and an easy, valveless venous return to convey the products of enzyme digestion back to the liver, for metabolic use. On evolutionary grounds it would seem probable that mesenteric flow would need to increase during digestion and decrease during exercise.

Most of what we surmise about the human being is based on animal experiments which are designed to measure pressure and flow in different parts of the bowel under varying conditions, and in particular to study the effects of acute ischaemia. Although, in spite of very different evolutionary influences, the basic pattern of blood supply to the intestine has remained fairly constant between mammalian species, the relevance of the animal data to man remains very difficult to determine, particularly as much of the experimental work has been carried out in dogs, whose splanchnic circulation is of a rather specialized design (see Chapter 2). (There is some evidence that the cat's visceral circulation is rather closer to our own.[40]) For ethical reasons, most of the methods available to the investigator in the animal laboratory cannot be used in clinical research.

At the time of writing there is no method of measuring blood flow to the intestine of a normal, intact resting or exercising man, and little prospect of knowing how this flow is shared between the different layers of the gut.

The remainder of this chapter is necessarily founded on information derived from animal work, but where an obvious discrepancy exists from what would be expected in human beings, this will be mentioned.

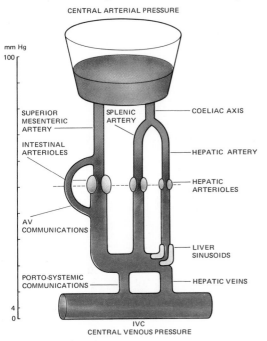

Fig. 3.1. The compartments of the splanchnic circulation, showing pressure relationships.

Methods of measuring intestinal blood flow

Qualitative methods

Simple observation of the colour of a loop of bowel, or of the arteries supplying it, gives a rough-and-ready guide to the adequacy of its nutrition, and in fact forms the basis of many crucial surgical decisions, in situations where exact measurements cannot be made. Likewise, the state of a mucosal circulation can be assessed by observing the colour of an accessible surface directly, endoscopically via a gastroscope or colonoscope, or by looking at a surgically constructed stoma.

The reliability of such simple tests is not very high, and it is difficult to judge by eye whether or not an ischaemic loop of bowel is able to recover.[15, 46] More accurate predictions can be made by measuring surface temperature during reactive hyperaemia or by recording action potentials from the muscle layers.[15] Although these methods do not measure absolute levels of flow, they are of use in estimating gross changes under different physiological circumstances, or following the administration of drugs.

Another technique (which has the (disadvantage of requiring a biopsy) equates blood flow with dehydrogenase activity by observing the time taken by a sample of tissue to reduce an injected dye such as tetrazolium bromide (MTT),[16] which appears to correlate with cell viability. This test works well in the laboratory but has yet to find a clinical application. A more recent refinement[59] has been the use of systemically injected [99M]Tc-labelled microspheres, which (theoretically at least) accumulate in the bowel in proportion to its blood flow, and can be detected there by normal counting methods. This gives good predictions of viability, and may prove to be of clinical use.

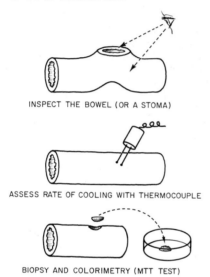

INSPECT THE BOWEL (OR A STOMA)

ASSESS RATE OF COOLING WITH THERMOCOUPLE

BIOPSY AND COLORIMETRY (MTT TEST)

Fig. 3.2. Estimation of intestinal blood flow—qualitative.

Quantitative methods

The direct method

The direct method of measuring total intestinal blood flow consisted simply in recording the output of the cannulated superior mesenteric vein (SMV) over a standard time, using a beaker and a stopwatch. The method is of historical interest and is only applicable to acute animal experiments; however, suitably modified, it forms the basis of an extremely accurate method of blood-flow measurement, in which the SMV output is passed in (calibrated) drops through silicon oil, recorded photoelectrically and returned to the animal. This is frequently used in academic physiology.[39]

Flowmeters.   These are of intravascular and extravascular types. The first variety operates on the principle of upstream and downstream pressure measurements (stromuhr) or of heat conduction (thermostromuhr), whereby a jet of fluid at known temperature is injected and recordings taken from a thermocouple inserted into the vessel at a standard distance below the site of injection. Such techniques are particularly useful in measuring low flow rates, as in the venous circulation, but of course the act of cannulation may introduce errors into the system.

These have largely been replaced by *extravascular flowmeters* based on ultrasonic or (more usually) electromagnetic principles, in which a probe is placed around the vessel and the current induced in the electromagnetic field by the moving stream of blood, amplified and then calibrated in terms of volume flow. Such probes can be implanted around the superior mesenteric artery and left in position for long periods, so that chronic experiments can be carried out,[12, 56] or responses in splanchnic flow to varying stimuli estimated in the conscious animal. In man, they have been used to measure flow during surgical operations, and are particularly useful in assessing the immediate result of an arterial reconstruction.[21] The main disadvantages of such flowmeters is the cost of having a sufficiently wide range of probe diameters to fit accurately around arteries of varying size, and the complexities involved in their calibration.

Clearance studies

Bromsulphthalein (BSP) and indocyanine green (ICG).   These have been used extensively in hepatic blood-flow measurements, using the Fick principle, as the hepatic veins are easily cannulated. Total hepatic blood flow closely approximates to total splanchnic flow, but of course gives little information regarding the intestinal component, due to the large and unpredictable contribution made by the hepatic artery and splenic vein. Because the superior mesenteric vein cannot be directly cannulated, it is not possible to use the method to measure intestinal flow in the intact animal. Measurements taken in this way[57] suggest that total splanchnic blood flow falls off sharply during exercise, which is at variance with flowmeter recordings from the SMA. If both methods are valid, this can only be explained on the basis of a massive drop in flow through the liver and spleen under exercise conditions, which does not seem particularly likely.

Amidopyrine.   Amidopyrine clearance has been used to measure gastric blood flow, as this substance appears to be secreted exclusively into the gastric juice. Labelled with ^{14}C it can also be used in the estimation of compartmental intestinal flow.[37, 40] It is too toxic for clinical use.

Isotope studies

External counting.   Absolon *et al.*[1] investigated the washout of intravenous ^{131}I by applying a Geiger counter to the abdominal wall at intervals following ligation of the superior mesenteric artery, and produced reproducible clearance curves. They were able to distinguish between the patent and the occluded SMA, but our own attempts to turn this to clinical use did not prove successful, because of the excessive background from the abdominal wall, the kidneys and retroperitoneal structures.[42]

Intraluminal recording.   A more refined modification is to introduce a Geiger–Muller (G–M) tube, enclosed in a plastic cylinder of known

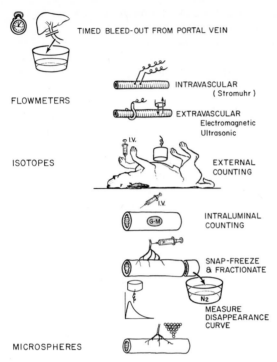

TIMED BLEED-OUT FROM PORTAL VEIN

FLOWMETERS

INTRAVASCULAR
(Stromuhr)

EXTRAVASCULAR
Electromagnetic
Ultrasonic

ISOTOPES

EXTERNAL
COUNTING

INTRALUMINAL
COUNTING

SNAP-FREEZE
& FRACTIONATE

MEASURE
DISAPPEARANCE
CURVE

MICROSPHERES

Fig. 3.3. Estimation of intestinal blood flow—quantitative.

diameter and thickness, into the intestinal lumen, and then to administer intravenously an isotope of known emittance and range such as ^{32}P.[4] This gives an indication of blood flow in the wall of the segment of intestine containing the counter but is at best semi-quantitative, first because as the isotope arrives in the gut wall as a 'wave' rather than a 'bolus', the washout curves are difficult to interpret, and secondly because ^{32}P acts as a non-diffusible isotope. In fact, the flows recorded in the human colon by this method are unexpectedly high. This may be due to inherent errors, but another possibility is that the G–M tube itself evokes a vasodilator reflex from the mucosa.[16, 17]

None the less the technique is non-invasive and applicable to man, and may well in the future provide quantitative data.

Intra-arterial injection techniques.   These techniques can be used to measure regional flow and also to study the distribution of blood flow between the different layers of the gut. A side-branch of a mesenteric vessel is cannulated and a slug of isotope (preferably a diffusing, fat-soluble substance such as ^{85}Kr) injected, while the gut is counted by detectors placed inside and outside the lumen. By using a scintillation counter to pick up γ activity and a G–M tube to detect β emission, an assessment can be made of total and muscularis flow, respectively[37] (see Fig. 3.4). This method is on the whole easier than detailed analysis of the washout curves.

Alternatively, a tracer such as ^{86}Rb is injected, the animal killed and snap-frozen and the radioactivity measured by autoradiography. Such experiments are, of course, acute and unrepeatable, and carry the objection that the uptake of a water-soluble isotope may not be directly flow-dependent.[40, 50]

Glass microspheres of diameter small enough to become arrested only in vessels of capillary size, and labelled with an isotope such as ^{24}Na, can be injected into an intestinal artery and the amount of isotope in each layer counted separately.[59] This method gives a high reading for submucosal flow as compared with other techniques, and again may not be totally reliable as microspheres tend to adhere to each other and form aggregates, and may adhere to the walls of the smaller vessels. Furthermore, there is some evidence of plasma skimming[34] in the mucosal circulation, and if the microsphere behaves as does a red blood cell, distribution will be uneven as the subepithelial blood is at a lower haematocrit.

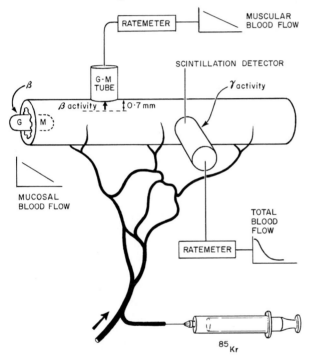

Fig. 3.4. Estimation of regional blood flow in the gut by isotope disappearance.

Total volume and flow

Measurement of total mesenteric blood volume in the dog is complicated by the presence of the spleen, which contracts in a rather unpredictable way in response to anaesthetic agents and surgical stress. It may contain as much as 10 per cent of the total blood volume, and furthermore this blood is of a haematocrit which is nearly twice the value found elsewhere, so that indicator dilution techniques are invalid, unless red cell volume and plasma volume are measured simultaneously and independently. Johnstone[36] used a technique of injecting ^{32}P-labelled red cells into the systemic circulation and, following a mixing period, isolating the viscera, and counting the contained radioactivity. He found the splanchnic blood volume to be some 20 per cent of the total, and this measurement has been amply confirmed since by other workers using other methods. Extrapolating these results to man, a 70 kg individual might be expected to have a total splanchnic blood volume in the region of 1,500 ml, though of course the splenic component of this would be much smaller than it is in the dog.

Total flow to the splanchnic bed was first estimated by the classical experiments of Burton-Opitz,[14] who inserted a stromuhr into the portal vein, and found a value of some 19 ml/kg per minute. The method was crude, but subsequent estimations have arrived at surprisingly similar values. The critical factors are the size of the animal, the blood pressure and the cardiac output, and when corrected for these variables total flow, as measured by portal bleed-out, stromuhr, isotope clearances[50, 51] and other methods, seems to be about 25 ml/kg per minute; that is to say, about 20 per cent of the cardiac output or 350–450 ml per minute in a 15 kg dog. When the components derived from stomach, pancreas and spleen are subtracted, this comes down to about 60 per cent of the total or 250 ml per minute.[26]

Applying these data to man gives a figure of 80–1,400 ml per minute, which accords well with direct observations made by application of an electromagnetic flowmeter to the superior mesenteric artery, during surgical operations.[21]

In other words, the intestinal blood volume and minute flow are roughly equivalent, so that this part of the circulation can be said to renew itself once every minute.

For obvious reasons, one would expect total flow to the alimentary tract to increase during digestion, and this is indeed what occurs. The classical stromuhr experiments of Herrick[30] showed that a standard meal raised flow in the superior mesenteric artery by 200 per cent, and that this was accompanied by increased flow in other vascular beds as well; that is to say, that hyperaemia within the gut was brought about not by diversion of blood from other organs but by a rise in cardiac output. These experiments were conducted under anaesthesia, and later work in conscious animals has produced rather different results.[12, 13, 56] Thus Burns and Schenk,[13] using implanted electromagnetic flowmeters, have shown that under fasting conditions the SMA takes 7·5 per cent of cardiac output but that this proportion doubles during digestion, without any rise in total output, suggesting that blood has been diverted from other organs. Measurements recorded during a meal show a slow rise of SMA flow to 50 per cent above normal, with no rise in cardiac output, whereas exercise causes a doubling in cardiac output with a 20 per cent fall in SMA flow.

There are two principal means whereby this 'digestive hyperaemia' is brought about. In the first place it has been shown by direct observation[10] and by cross-circulation experiments[22] that the gastrointestinal hormones (gastrin, secretin, cholecystokinin) whose release is stimulated by the presence of food in the duodenum, all increase flow in the SMA. Secondly, the local nervous reflex referred to below, in which contact between the mucosa and the contents of the lumen induce local vasodilatation, is clearly important.

Regulation of flow

The factors which determine the volume of blood reaching the intestine per unit time, and the way in which it is distributed throughout the intestinal wall, are complex and interdependent. If they are to be studied at all they have necessarily to be measured in isolation from each other, and it must be admitted that much of the work in this subject has an air of artificiality about it, and is of doubtful validity in the context of the intact working body. The more important determinants of intestinal blood flow are set out in schematic form in Figs. 3.1, 3.5 and 3.6.

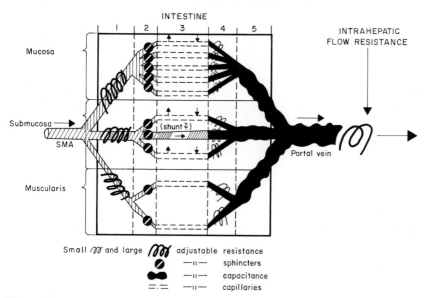

Fig. 3.5. Vascular resistances in the intestinal wall. (Reproduced from *Gastroenterology* (1967), **52**, 423–431, by courtesy of Professor B. Folkow and the Editor.)

Centrally determined factors

These comprise the cardiac output, the central arterial pressure and the blood viscosity.

Mesenteric blood flow clearly will depend on the output of the *left ventricle* and, in fact, falls to half during each diastolic cycle.[32] With a prolonged fall in cardiac output the intestinal circulation tends to behave as a 'low priority area', so that the arterioles shut down and flow drops off. This has relevance to the occurrence of gut necrosis as a complication of hypotension and 'shock', and to the concept of non-occlusive intestinal infarction, which is discussed further, below.

The *arterial blood pressure* is a function of the cardiac output and of the total peripheral resistance, of which the intestinal resistance is a part. Vasodilatation in other vascular beds will reduce both central pressure and mesenteric blood flow, but this effect is to some extent mitigated by the mechanism of autoregulation.

Autoregulation of a vascular bed implies its capacity to maintain, by internal compensations, a constant blood flow in the face of fluctuations in central arterial pressure (in this case, in the SMA). This means that rises in SMA pressure lead to constriction of, and falls to dilatation of, the precapillary resistance vessels. The arterioles seem normally to operate with their smooth muscle in a state of partial contraction; in other words, with a set level of 'resting tone' which can be relaxed or intensified.[25] This tone is the result of a balance between the opposing forces which are shown in Fig. 3.6. The role of the sympathetic and of circulating pressor substances is complex. While locally released or circulating adrenaline causes initial contraction of the arteriolar muscle of an isolated loop preparation, this is not maintained for more than a few minutes, and the effect then becomes one of vasodilatation (autoregulatory escape). The action of noradrenaline, however, is almost purely vasoconstrictor.[54] The exact way in which these agents interact in the organ as a whole, and the differing effects of local or systemic administration, are far from being understood (see below).

The effects of lowering or raising arterial pressure are, however, more clear-cut. Artificial lowering of the pressure produces an immediate fall in flow and rise in resistance which is followed after a few seconds by compensatory return towards the original level. The initial reduction in flow is clearly due to the fall in arteriovenous pressure difference, and the increase in resistance to the elastic recoil of the vessel wall.[25] The secondary changes cannot be due to a reduction in blood viscosity (as this increases with low flow rates) so must be due to dilatation of the resistance vessels. This has been observed direct in the mesenteric circulation of the cat[35] using the flying spot microscope technique. Moderate alterations in pressure are almost immediately compensated so as to maintain normal flow, but clearly the autoregulating process can only operate within defined limits. When the pressure is lowered to a level at which the arteriolar muscle is completely relaxed (about 60 mm Hg) then further falls will cause diminution in vessel calibre with consequent increase in resistance and fall in flow, until such point as the vessel collapses completely and flow ceases (the disputed 'critical closing pressure'). At these very low flow rates the process of vasodilatation is augmented and hastened by the accumulation of vasoactive metabolites,[55] but it seems that at high or normal flow rates the myogenic response is capable of overcoming this effect. Thus if the venous pressure is raised, thus simultaneously reducing tissue pO_2 and pH and raising intravascular pressure, there is an immediate and sharp rise in vascular resistance and fall in flow.

The *blood viscosity* depends on many variables, the most influential of which is the haematocrit. Haemoconcentration from any cause will tend to decrease intestinal blood flow. This mechanism operates particularly in acute intestinal ischaemia, which results in massive plasma loss with a rapid rise in local and total blood viscosity.[41] The finer regulation of viscosity, dependent on fibrinogen levels and shear rates along irregular vessel walls, has not so far been shown to have clinical importance in the mesenteric circulation.

The sympathetic nervous system

It is conveniently supposed that sympathetic activity constricts arterioles and decreases blood flow in the skin and gut, but this oversimplifies what happens. Stimulation of splanchnic nerves produces an immediate rise in mesenteric vascular resistance and fall in flow, presumably due to stimulation of α receptors. However, when the stimulus is continued there is a gradual return of flow towards normal levels, which is eventually followed by vascular relaxation and hyperaemia.[53] This 'autoregulatory escape' is not clearly understood but may be related partly to the relaxation in smooth muscle tone in the gut wall brought about by sympathetic stimulation, and partly to the accumulation of vasodilatory metabolites in the ischaemic tissue. There are no parasympathetic vasodilator fibres in the small bowel[38] (though there may well be some in the colon, arriving via the sacral autonomic nerves[31] and if there are β receptors in the intestinal wall they are probably not innervated. In any event, the effect of parasympathetic activity would be to increase smooth muscle tone in the intestinal wall, which would itself tend to limit flow.

As would be expected, section of the splanchnic nerves results in vascular dilatation and a fall in resistance.

'Humoral' mechanisms

This rather dated phraseology has been deliberately chosen, in order to encompass a broad range of substances (enzymes, hormones, neurotrans-

Table 3.1. Vasoactive agents in the splanchnic circulation

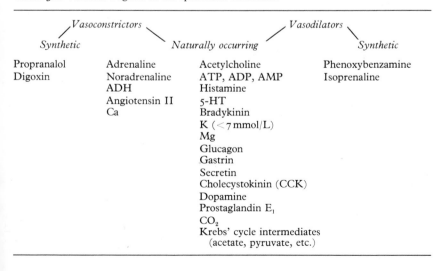

Vasoconstrictors		Vasodilators	
Synthetic	*Naturally occurring*		*Synthetic*
Propranalol	Adrenaline	Acetylcholine	Phenoxybenzamine
Digoxin	Noradrenaline	ATP, ADP, AMP	Isoprenaline
	ADH	Histamine	
	Angiotensin II	5-HT	
	Ca	Bradykinin	
		K ($<7\,$mmol/L)	
		Mg	
		Glucagon	
		Gastrin	
		Secretin	
		Cholecystokinin (CCK)	
		Dopamine	
		Prostaglandin E$_1$	
		CO_2	
		Krebs' cycle intermediates (acetate, pyruvate, etc.)	

mitters and products of metabolism), not all of which have been positively identified but which influence blood flow in the alimentary tract independently of intact nervous pathways.

1. Transmitter substances

(i) **Adrenaline and noradrenaline** are secreted by the adrenal medulla and released from postganglionic sympathetic nerves. Their concentration at the point of action thus depends on the level of sympathetic drive and on medullary activity. But the effect of experimental intra-arterial injection of these substances is, from all reported sources, quite unpredictable. Adrenaline, for example, has been variously reported to increase and decrease resistance in the mesenteric vascular bed.[3, 26, 32, 54] Its effect on the veins appears to depend on intravenous pressure, as it increases distensibility over the range of 15–30 mm Hg, but decreases compliance at 7–11 mm Hg. This apparent paradox probably reflects the particular receptor which is activated; adrenaline administered at a low infusion rate appears to act selectively on β receptors, but when the level is raised vasoconstriction results from a preponderance of α stimulating activity. Pretreatment with α blockers such as phenoxybenzamine results in a dilator response to adrenaline. Additionally, the direct metabolic effect of the amine on carbohydrate metabolism, which may result in the production of vasodilator metabolites, and its effect on the tone of the smooth muscle of the gut wall, cannot be ignored.[27] When given into a systemic vein, adrenaline raises the level of SMA flow, presumably due to selective vasoconstriction in other vascular compartments.

Noradrenaline when given into a local artery produces vasoconstriction. Given systemically, it usually produces constriction, though later autoregulatory escape may occur.[27] Whatever its local effects, noradrenaline will in general raise the blood pressure, slow the heart and decrease cardiac output, thus diminishing over-all mesenteric blood flow.

(ii) **Acetylcholine,** infused intra-arterially at a low level, produces vasodilatation in the intestinal vascular bed. Larger quantities may, however, increase gastrointestinal motility with a simultaneous rise in resistance and decline in flow.[3]

(iii) **Dopamine** given intravenously raises arterial blood pressure and aortic, renal and superior mesenteric arterial flow. It appears to be a potent vasodilator of the intestinal vascular bed, acting on both α and β receptors and also perhaps on others, as yet unidentified, which are blocked by the administration of apomorphine.[21, 44] Dopamine probably acts physiologically by inhibiting prolactin release, and work by Muriuki *et al.*[47] on rats suggests that although prolactin has no direct constrictor effect on the mesenteric circulation it is capable of antagonizing the pressor effects of noradrenaline.

(iv) **Histamine.** Present in the Paneth cells in the gut wall and in the circulating blood, histamine also has an erratic effect on the mesenteric circulation. Injected into the superior mesenteric artery the usual response is vasodilatation, but if large quantities are administered its central effect on blood pressure becomes predominant and mesenteric flow falls off.

2. Hormones

(i) **5-Hydroxytryptamine** (5-HT). This is present in high concentration in the mucosa of the gastrointestinal tract.[49] When given intra-arterially, it can produce either a decrease, no change or an increase in gastrointestinal blood flow, depending on the relative importance of its effect on vascular and visceral smooth muscle. In the main, the effect is to shift the site of resistance from the small to the large vessels, thus diminishing the tone of the precapillary resistance.

(ii) **Antidiuretic hormone** (ADH, vasopressin). This is the most potent naturally occurring vasoconstrictor in the mesenteric circulation.[54] Intravenously, it produces an abrupt reduction of blood flow in the SMA and portal vein together with contraction of the spleen. This effect has been put to clinical use in the treatment of bleeding oesophageal varices.[5]

(iii) **Angiotensin II.** This has a similar constricting effect on the whole of the splanchnic vasculature.

(iv) **Kinins.** Both bradykinin and kallidin are potent vasodilators to the intestinal arteries, and when given intra-arterially produce a profound drop in vascular resistance throughout the alimentary tract.

(v) **Glucagon.** This has a similar dilatory effect, and at the same time has been shown to relax the smooth muscle of both the small and the large intestine.[45] This, coupled with its inotropic action, makes it a very promising agent for use in low-flow states involving the gut. Glucagon has, in fact, already found some application in intestinal angiography,[18] where it has been shown to improve the quality of image, by permitting contrast material to permeate small vessels. It has the disadvantage of causing quite pronounced nausea when given in an effective dose. These actions of glucagon are pharmacological rather than physiological, and whether in fact the small concentration present in the splanchnic blood during life has any physiological role to play must remain doubtful.

(vi) **Gastrin, secretin and cholecystokinin (CCK).** As already mentioned, all these increase SMA flow. Release of these hormones is stimulated by the presence of food in the duodenum, and they undoubtedly play an important part in raising blood flow in the alimentary tract during the digestive process.

(vii) **Prostaglandins.** There is some evidence that prostaglandin E_1 has a similar effect to glucagon on the splanchnic circulation, and work on dogs[19] has demonstrated a doubling of SMA flow when doses of between

0·01 and 1·0 mg/kg are given intravenously. This effect has also been suggested as being of potential clinical use in gastrointestinal angiography.

(viii) **Metabolites.**   (*a*) In perfusion experiments, a rise in pCO_2 in the perfusate causes a rise in SMA flow, whereas variations in pH while the pCO_2 is kept constant appear to produce no change. This dilator effect of CO_2 is also seen after adrenergic blockade, whereas the response to adrenaline is greater at low than at high pH.[43] Similar dilator effects have been noted from the intra-arterial infusion of ATP, ADP, AMP, pyruvate, acetate, citrate, fumarate and other intermediate products of the Krebs cycle.[27]

(*b*) Increased concentration of *potassium ion* appears to exert a biphasic effect on the mesenteric vasculature. When the concentration is at about 4 mmol/litre vasodilatation occurs, but with progressive rises to above 10 mmol/litre this is succeeded by vasoconstriction. This effect appears to be closely related to the influence of the ion on intestinal wall tension.[48] An interesting corollary here is that increases in intestinal motility, or in distension of the gut wall, both cause increased potassium concentration in the portal venous blood, which may be responsible for the compensatory vasodilatation.

The effect of magnesium appears to be wholly dilatory, whereas calcium is predominantly a vasoconstrictor.[54]

3. Local mechanical factors

(i) **Resistances in the gut wall.** Arterial resistance (Fig. 3.6) is a function of length as well as of radius. Alterations in the disposition of a loop of intestine may lengthen or shorten the course of the vessels in the mesentery and gut wall, and correspondingly increase or decrease their resistance to flow. The spiral, tortuous arrangement of many of the splanchnic arteries compensates partially for this effect. Additionally, the tone of the smooth muscle of the gut exerts an important 'squeeze' effect on the intramural vessels (Fig. 3.6).

Folkow[23] has described the circulation of the intestinal wall as consisting of a number of vascular circuits running in parallel, with resistances in series (see Fig. 3.5).

The precapillary resistance section comprises the arteriolar sphincters which here, as in most other parts of the body, are the chief determinant of the peripheral resistance. To this must be added the 'squeeze' effect of the muscle of the gut wall, which has an important effect in limiting flow. The presence of the muscular and submucosal plexuses, which allow free communication of blood between adjoining segments, to an extent mitigates this effect, and equalizes flow between adjacent segments of bowel.

The capillary exchange section is most developed in the crypts and villi, and though crucial for effective absorptive and excretory function plays a rather lesser role in the regulation of blood flow, as changes in this area are largely passive. Blood emerging from this section is subject to *postcapillary resistances* exerted by venular sphincters (and by the gut wall) and

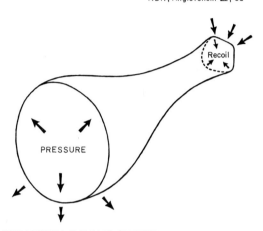

FACTORS WHICH REDUCE DIAMETER

MECHANICAL   Elastic Recoil
              Muscular 'Squeeze'
              Abdominal Pressure

NERVOUS   Sympathetic (Short acting)

HUMORAL   Adrenaline, Noradrenaline
              ADH, Angiotensin II, Ca

Recoil

PRESSURE

FACTORS WHICH INCREASE DIAMETER

MECHANICAL   Hydrostatic Pressure

NERVOUS   Sympathetic (long acting)

HUMORAL CO_2 Lactate. Krebs cycle
              Intermediates Mg

Fig. 3.6. Factors affecting the diameter of the intestinal arteriole.

finally enters the *venous capacitance section* which contains the greater part of the splanchnic blood volume and runs at low pressure and low velocity. There are no valves in the portal system of veins, so that the final resistance, which is that of the liver sinusoid, acts unimpeded on the venous drainage of the bowel. The physical characteristics of the arterial wall have an important bearing on the elastic recoil which it exerts on the blood stream, and on its capacity to alter its diameter in the face of changing circumstances. Naturally occurring obstructive lesions are usually found at the origins of three main vessels, and affect flow at the periphery in an indirect way. In fact, the intermediate and minute vessels do not appear to change very much with age, and their mechanical properties do not seem to be of great clinical importance. However, there is some evidence[52] that in arterial hypertension the intestinal arteries are significantly narrowed due to medial contracture, in the absence of any significant intimal thickening.

(ii) **Local reflexes.**   Friction on the mucosa produces local vasodilatation.[6] This effect is independent of central nervous pathways and is not an axon reflex because it is not abolished by chronic denervation.[6] The exact mechanism by which the effect is produced is unknown, but it appears to be mediated via an intramural reflex arc involving 5-HT receptors. The same reflex appears to be stimulated by hypertonic glucose instilled into the lumen.[17] It must be remembered that the insorptive and exsorptive work of the intestine and the production of vasoactive metabolites occur at the end of the villus; that is to say, at an area far removed from the control of blood flow, which is determined by resistance vessels. As was pointed out in Chapter 2, the arteriole loses its muscular coat about one-third of the way up the villus, so that the luminal area is in a sense defenceless against fluctuations in input pressure.

There is an additional significance to the local reflex, in that any technique of blood-flow measurement which relies on a device having contact with the mucosa may invoke this response.

(iii) **The effect of distension.** Boley[9] studied the effects of increased intraluminal pressure on blood flow through the wall of the dog's colon, using a flowmeter on the afferent artery and [85]Kr washout curves from the mucosa. They found little change until the intraluminal pressure was above 30 mm Hg, at which point a sharp drop occurred to levels of 20–35 per cent of normal. Injection studies and [85]Kr washout curves suggested that flow falls off initially in the mucosa.

These findings have important clinical bearings on the association between intestinal obstruction and ischaemic damage (see Chapter 8).

Distribution of flow within the gut wall

It is generally true that blood flow through an organ is related to its demands for oxygen, and such is the case with the smooth muscle of the gut, whose consumption is in fact quite low. However, in the case of the villi and the crypts which are concerned, respectively, with the absorption and secretion of material, the volume of blood required is related not only to oxygen demand but also to the need for fluid transport, as the plasma is the vehicle which conducts material into and out of the lumen. The inner layers of the gut thus have a much higher blood flow than their oxygen requirements alone would warrant, and there exists a system of internal switching mechanisms which redistributes flow from one layer to another, even while total blood flow remains constant.

Most of our knowledge of the intimate behaviour of the small bowel circulation comes from the work of Folkow and his fellow workers in Göteborg. It was he who developed the concept of parallel and serial coupling of the vascular resistances within the gut wall which was described above.[23]

Although the capillaries are the crucial area in that the secretion of mucus and enzymes and the absorption of nutriments take place across their membranes, they themselves play little or no part in the regulation of flow, but rather accept what they are given. The number and distribution of open capillaries is regulated by the precapillary sphincters, but the total amount of blood available is determined by the arterioles, which constitute the main resistance. The intracapillary pressure, and hence the shift of fluid in and out of the vessels, is determined by the gradient between the arteriolar and venular ends, so that the tone of the venules, which is strongly influenced by the neural and chemical regulators described above, has an influence here.

Experiments designed to study the distribution of blood flow to the different layers of the gut using water-soluble isotopes such as ^{86}Rb may be misleading in that extraction of the material by the tissues is probably incomplete except at very low rates of flow. Lundgren[7, 8, 28, 34, 39, 40] has overcome these objections using lipid-soluble gases such as [85]Kr, whose clearance is flow-dependent. By studying the washout curves of this isotope following local and intravascular injection, and examining autoradiographs after injection of antipyrine–[14]C, he concludes that four zones of the small intestinal wall can be distinguished, each with a characteristic rate of clearance.

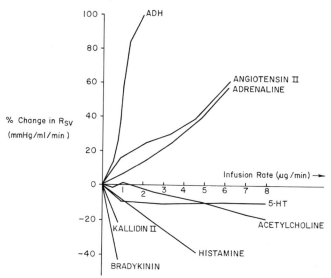

Fig. 3.7. Action of vasomotor substances on intestinal blood flow. (Modified, by kind permission, from E. Clinton Texter *et al.*, 1968, *Physiology of the Gastrointestinal Tract*; St. Louis, C. V. Mosley Co.)

It will be noted that under resting conditions total flow amounts to 30–35 ml/100 g tissue per minute, rising to 200–250 ml/kg per minute when maximum vasodilatation is induced with isopropylnoradrenaline.[6, 7] Most of the blood goes to the mucosa, which has flow rate about three times that of the muscle, but there exists in the deeper part of the crypts and in the submucosa a region of exceptionally high vascularity of some 400–600 ml/100 g per minute. With vasodilatation, there was a redistribution of flow in favour of this area, which now takes 50–60 per cent of the total, at flow rates of 800–1,000 ml/100 g tissue per minute.

In later studies Jodal and Lundgren,[33, 34] using ^{51}Cr-labelled red cells and ^{125}I-labelled albumin, have confirmed that a large fraction of the regional blood volume is to be found in this submucosal and deep mucosal layer, perhaps because this is where the veins are concentrated. The total blood contained in the deep mucosa and submucosa of the small gut is about the same as that within the liver. However, on a unit weight basis the submucosa of the small intestine seems to contain about twice as much blood as does that of the colon, perhaps due to the relatively greater proportion of submucosal tissue in the large bowel. The presence of a highly vascular layer of bowel wall in the deep mucosa is perhaps to be expected, as not only is this an area of high secretory activity, but also it is here that the new epithelium is manufactured.

The intestinal countercurrent exchanger

Isotope studies[39, 40] demonstrate that during resting conditions, and to a rather lesser extent during absorption or following vasodilatation, there is a fast-moving component of the clearance curve, which appears to clear more rapidly than could be expected if the whole capillary network had been traversed, and may represent direct arteriovenous shunting. The existence of anatomical and physiological arteriovenous connections in the intestinal wall has been disputed for many years (see Chapter 1). Though Spanner was confident of their presence in the villus of man and the submucosa of the dog, subsequent authors[11] have failed to demonstrate them except in small numbers, and microsphere injection studies[58] suggest that the total 'shunt-flow' in the dog is not more than 3–4 per cent of the total. It seems unlikely that movement of whole blood from artery to vein could account for the discrepancy.

The 'hairpin' arrangement of vessels in the villus (see Fig. 2.11), with the afferent and efferent vessels running close together in opposite directions, is reminiscent of that in the nephron where countercurrent exchange has been shown to take place, and it has been thought possible that a similar mechanism is at work in the intestine. Evidence is accumulating that this is in fact the case. For a detailed discussion of this the reader is referred to the work of Lundgren,[40] but some of the main points are as follows:

1. Oxygen clears faster than do labelled red cells when injected intra-arterially, suggesting extravascular shunting.

2. The expected 'delay' effect of a countercurrent exchanger, which operates through the presence of a reversed concentration gradient at the base of the villus, is seen following injection of ^{85}Kr. A Geiger–Muller counter within the lumen registers a slow continuous increase of activity as the isotope becomes redistributed within the villus.

3. When flow is raised to above 150 ml/100 g per minute, these findings no longer obtain. This would be expected, as countercurrent exchange across a hairpin loop falls off proportional to the linear velocity along the loop.

If such a countercurrent exchange mechanism exists (and there is evidence from other sources that it does) then it must have a profound importance on intestinal function. The transfer of a solute into the venous blood of the villus will create an arteriovenous concentration gradient, so that a fraction of the solute will diffuse into the central artery and be conducted back to the tip of the villus. This creates a zone of hyperosmolarity at the tip of the villus, which can be demonstrated by cryoscopic techniques.

The net effect of this will be to delay absorption of lipophilic substances, and the degree of delay will depend on the anatomy of the villus, the permeability of the vascular walls, the linear velocity of blood in the vessel and the diffusion characteristics of the solute, bearing in mind that the transit time in the arteriole is about one-tenth that in the capillaries and venules.

This delaying device has an obvious physiological usefulness in the protection of the intravascular compartment from abrupt rises in osmolarity (Fig. 3.8a), and may assist in the absorption of water.

The exchanger might also be expected to protect against loss of material

(a)   (b)

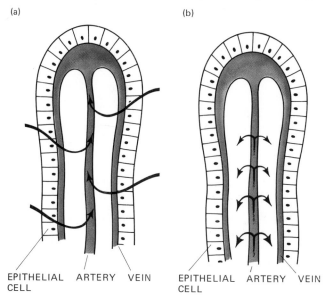

EPITHELIAL   ARTERY   VEIN   EPITHELIAL   ARTERY   VEIN
CELL   CELL

Fig. 3.8 (a and b). The intestinal countercurrent exchange mechanism.

of small molecular weight from the circulation into the lumen of the bowel, where there is a major difference in arterial and venous concentration of the solute. Extravascular shunting will then progressively increase the venous concentration at the base of the villus, preventing a high concentration in the capillaries of the tip, whence loss could occur into the lumen (Fig. 3.8b).

Finally, the mechanism is of the utmost importance in ischaemia, where progressive reduction in linear velocity of the blood, resulting from fall in input pressure and increase in viscosity, will lead to shunting of oxygen across the base of the villus, thus depriving the tip and causing ulceration,[2, 28, 29] or the separation of a pseudomembrane. This will be discussed in detail in Chapter 5.

References

1   Absolon, K. B., Long, V. and Hunter, S. W. (1960). An experimental study of the diagnosis of Mesenteric Infarction. *Surgery, Gynecology and Obstetrics* **110:** 617–620.

2 Ahren, C. and Haglund, U. (1973). Mucosal lesions in the small intestine of the cat during low flow. *Acta Physiologica Scandinavica* **88**: 1–9.

3 Appel, A. J., Lintermans, J. P., Mullins, G. L. and Guntheroth, W. G. (1966). The effects of vasoactive drugs on mesenteric blood flow and volume. *Surgery, Gynecology and Obstetrics* **123**: 755–764.

4 Bacaner, M. B. and Pollycove, M. (1962) Determination in vivo of regional circulatory dynamics in intact intestine. *American Journal of Physiology* **203**: 1094–1102.

5 Baum, S. and Nusbaum, M. (1971). The control of gastrointestinal haemorrhage by selective mesenteric arterial infusion of vasopressin. *Vascular Disorders of the Intestine*, pp. 459–471. Ed. by S. J. Boley. New York and London, Appleton-Century-Crofts.

6 Biber, B., Lundgren, D. and Svanvik, J. (1971). Studies on the intestinal vasodilatation observed after mechanical stimulation of the mucosa of the gut. *Acta Physiologica Scandinavica* **82**: 177–190.

7 Biber, B., Lundgren, O. and Svanvik, J. (1973). Intramural blood-flow and blood volume in the small intestine of the cat as analysed by an indicator dilution technique. *Acta Physiologica Scandinavica* **87**: 391–403.

8 Biber, V., Lundgren, O., Stage, L. and Svanvik, J. (1973). An indicator dilution method for studying intestinal hemodynamics in the cat. *Acta Physiologica Scandinavica* **87**: 433–447.

9 Boley, S. J., Agrawal, G., Warren, A., Veith, F. J., Levowits, B. S., Treiber, W., Dougherty, J., Schwartz, S. S. and Gliedman, M. H. (1969). Pathophysiologic effects of bowel distension on intestinal blood-flow. *American Journal of Surgery* **117**: 228–234.

10 Bowen, J. C., Pawlik, W., Fang, W. F. and Jacobson, E. D. (1975) Pharmacologic effects of gastrointestinal hormones on intestinal oxygen consumption and blood flow. *Surgery* **78**: 515–519.

11 Brockis, J. G. and Moffat, D. B. (1958). The intrinsic blood vessels of the pelvic colon. *Journal of Anatomy* **92**: 52–56.

12 Burns, G. P. and Schenk, W. G. (1967). Intestinal blood-flow in the conscious dog. *Surgical Forum* **18**: 313–315.

13 Burns, G. P. and Schenk, W. G. (1969). Effect of digestion and exercise on intestinal blood flow and cardiac output. *Archives of Surgery* **98**: 790–794.

14 Burton-Opitz, R. (1911). The vascularity of the liver. IV. The magnitude of the portal inflow. *Quarterly Journal of Experimental Physiology* **4**: 113–117.

15 Bussemaker, J. B. and Lindeman, J. (1972). Comparison of methods to determine viability of small intestine. *Annals of Surgery* **176**: 97–101.

16 Carter, K., Halle, M., Cherry, G. and Myers, M. B. (1970). Determination of the viability of ischaemic intestine. *Archives of Surgery* **100**: 695–701.

17 Chou, C. C., Burns, T. D., Hsieh, C. P. and Dabney, J. M. (1972). Mechanisms of local vasodilation with hypertonic glucose in the jejunum. *Surgery* **71**: 380–387.

18 Danford, R. O. and Davidson, A. J. (1969). The use of glucagon as a vasodilator in visceral angiography. *Radiology* **93**: 173–175.

19 Davis, W., Anderson, J. H., Wallace, S., Gianturco, C. and Jacobson, E. D. (1975). The use of prostaglandin E¹ to enhance the angiographic visualization of the splanchnic circulation. *Radiology* **114**: 281–286.

20 Dawson, A. M., Trenchard, D. and Guz, A. (1965). Small bowel tonometry—assessment of small gut mucosal oxygen tension in dog and man. *Nature* **206**: 943–944.

21 Edwards, A. J. and Taylor, G. (1970). Experience with the coeliac axis compression syndrome. *British Medical Journal* **1**: 342–345.

22 Fara, J. W., Rubinstein, E. H. and Sonnenschein, R. R. (1972). Intestinal hormones in mesenteric vasodilation after intraduodenal agents. *American Journal of Physiology* **223**: 1058–1067.
23 Folkow, B. (1967). Regional adjustments of intestinal blood-flow. *Gastroenterology* **52**: 423–431.
24 Goldberg, L. I. (1972). Cardiovascular and renal actions of dopamine: potential clinical applications. *Pharmacological Reviews* **24**: 1–29.
25 Gore, R. W. (1974). Pressures in cat mesenteric arterioles and capillaries during changes in systemic arterial blood pressure. *Circulation Research* **34**: 581–591.
26 Grim, E. (1963). The flow of blood in the mesenteric vessels. *Handbook of Physiology*, Vol. 11, *Circulation* 1439–1456. Washington, DC, American Physiological Society.
27 Haddy, F. J., Chou, C. C., Scott, J. B. and Dabney, J. M. (1967) Intestinal vascular response to naturally occurring vasoactive substances. *Gastroenterology* **52**: 444–450.
28 Haglund, U. and Lundgren, O. (1974). The small intestine in haemorrhagic shock. *Gastroenterology* **66**: 625–627.
29 Haglund, U., Hulten, L., Aksen, C. and Lundgren, O. (1976). Mucosal lesions in the human small intestine in shock. *Gut* **16**: 929–984.
30 Herrick, J. F., Essex, H. E., Mann, F. C. and Baldes, E. J. (1934). The effect of digestion on blood-flow in certain blood vessels of the dog. *American Journal of Physiology* **108**: 621–628.
31 Hultén, L. (1969). Extrinsic nervous control of colonic motility and blood flow. *Acta Physiologica Scandinavica*, Suppl. 335.
32 Jacobson, E. D. (1971). Physiologic aspects of the intestinal circulation. In: *Vascular Disorders of the Intestine*, p. 20. Ed. by S. J. Boley. New York and London, Appleton-Century-Crofts.
33 Jodal, M. and Lundgren, O. (1970). Regional distribution of red cells, plasma and blood volume in the intestinal wall of the cat. *Acta Physiologica Scandinavica* **80**: 533–537.
34 Jodal, M. and Lundgren, O. (1970). Plasma skimming in the intestinal tract. *Acta Physiologica Scandinavica* **80**: 50–60.
35 Johnson, P. C. (1968). Autoregulatory responses of cat mesenteric arterioles measured in vivo. *Circulation Research* **22**: 199–205.
36 Johnstone, F. R. C. (1956). Measurement of splanchnic blood volume in dogs. *American Journal of Physiology* **185**: 450–452.
37 Kampp, M., Lundgren, O. and Sjostrand, J. (1968). On the components of the Kr 85 washout curves from the small intestine of the cat. *Acta Physiologica Scandinavica* **72**: 257–281.
38 Kewenter, J. (1965). The vagal control of the jejunal and ileal motility and blood-flow. *Acta Physiologica Scandinavica* **65**: Suppl. 251, 1–68.
39 Lundgren, O. (1967). Studies on blood-flow distribution and countercurrent exchange in the small intestine. *Acta Physiologica Scandinavica*, Suppl. 303.
40 Lundgren, O. (1974). The circulation of the small bowel mucosa. *Gut* **15**: 1005–1013.
41 Marston, A. (1963). Causes of death in mesenteric arterial occlusion. *Annals of Surgery* **158**: 952–959.
42 Marston, A. and Gimlette, T. M. D. (1962). Unpublished observations.
43 McGinn, F. D., Mendel, D. and Perry, D. M. (1967). The effects of alteration of CO_2 and pH on intestinal blood-flow in the cat. *Journal of Physiology* **192**: 669–680.
44 Merlo, L. and Marchetti, G. (1974). Azioni vasodilatrice della dopamina sui vasi renali e mesenteriche dopo blocco adrenergico α e β. *Bolletino della Societa Italiana di Biologia Sperimentale* **50**: 1584–1590.

45   Merrill, S. L., Chvojka, V. E., Berkowitz, G. M. and Texter, E. C. (1962) The effect of glucagon on the superior mesenteric vascular bed. *Federation Proceedings* **21**: 200–205.

46   Moossa, A. R., Skinner, D. B., Stark, V. and Hoffer, P. (1974). Assessment of bowel viability using 99^m technetium-tagged albumen microspheres. *Journal of Surgical Research* **16**: 466–472.

47   Muriuki, P. B., Mugambi, M., Thairu, K., Mathai, S. and Mati, J. K. G. (1974). The effects of prolactin on the responses of the isolated mesenteric artery of the rat to noradrenaline. *East African Medical Journal* **51**: 232–235.

48   Nelson, R. A. and Beargie, R. J. (1965). The effect of reduced arterial pressure and flow on intestinal function. *Surgery, Gynecology and Obstetrics* **120**: 1221–1224.

49   Resnick, R. H. and Gray, S. J. (1961). Distribution of serotonin (5-hydroxytryptamine) in the human gastrointestinal tract. *Gastroenterology* **41**: 2–7.

50   Sapirstein, L. A. (1958). Regional blood-flow by fractional distribution of indicators. *American Journal of Physiology* **193**: 151–168.

51   Selkurt, E. E. and Wathen, R. L. (1967) Washout of intra-arterially injected xenon 133 from the intestine of the dog as a method for estimating blood-flow. *Gastroenterology* **52**: 387–390.

52   Short, D. S. and Thomson, A. D. (1959). The intestinal arteries in hypertension. *Journal of Pathology and Bacteriology* **78**: 321–325.

53   Svanvik, J. (1973). Mucosal hemodynamics in the small intestine of the cat during regional sympathetic vasoconstrictor activation. *Acta Physiologica Scandinavica* **89**: 19–29.

54   Texter, E. C., Chou, C. C., Laureta, H. C. and Vantrappen, G. R. (1968). *Physiology of the Gastrointestinal Tract*. St Louis, Mo., C. V. Mosby Co.

55   Turner, M. D., Neely, W. A. and Barnett, W. O. (1959). Effects of arterial, venous and arteriovenous occlusion on intestinal blood-flow. *Surgery, Gynecology and Obstetrics* **108**, 347–351.

56   Vatner, S. F., Franklin, D. and van Citters, R. L. (1970). Mesenteric vasoactivity associated with eating and digestion in the conscious dog. *American Journal of Physiology* **219**: 170–174.

57   Wade, O. L., Combes, B., Childs, A. W., Wheeler, H. O., Cournand, A. and Bradley, S. E. (1956). The effect of exercise on splanchnic blood flow and splanchnic blood volume in normal man. *Clinical Science* **15**: 547–552.

58   Yu, Y. M., Yu, C. C. L. and Chou, C. C. (1975). Distribution of blood-flow in the intestine with hypertonic glucose in the lumen. *Surgery* **78**: 520–525.

59   Zarins, C. K., Skinner, D. B. and James, A. E. (1974). Prediction of the viability of devascularized intestine with radioactive microspheres. *Surgery, Gynecology and Obstetrics* **138**: 576–579.

4

Laboratory Studies of Intestinal Ischaemia

Introduction

It is very easy to interfere with the arterial supply to the intestine in the experimental laboratory, and there exists a large body of information as to methods and results. Thus ligation of the SMA and later release of the ligature has been used for years as a standard shock model, the ischaemic loop preparation is the recognized model for the study of strangulation-obstruction, and chronic occlusion by means of Ameroid cylinders has shed some light on the pathophysiology of chronic ischaemia.

Because, however, of different patterns of evolution of the alimentary tract, there are enormous species differences in the behaviour of the ischaemic intestine, so that great care must be taken when extrapolating animal data to human beings. This particularly applies to the role played by the splanchnic circulation in shock and low-flow states.

The three principal techniques which have been used in the study of the ischaemic bowel are:

1. Acute occlusion of the SMA, with or without subsequent release.
2. Chronic obliteration of the main arteries.
3. Occlusion of the IMA and the smaller segmental vessels.

These will be discussed individually.

Acute occlusion of the superior mesenteric artery

Effects on the bowel

The effects of ligation of the superior mesenteric artery have now been studied for over a hundred years, as 1975 marked the centenary of Litten's original experiments.[44]

He found that ligation of the artery in 40 dogs resulted in every case in death within 12–48 hours, accompanied by vomiting, bloody diarrhoea and fever.

The immediate effects of tying the SMA were as follows. All pulsations disappeared, the bowel became blue-white and spastic, with collapsed arteries and prominent veins. Contractions initially increased, but eventually disappeared, and after some hours the loops became relaxed and distended. After 8–10 hours frank haemorrhage began to occur and finally at autopsy the bowel from the duodenojejunal flexure to the transverse colon was dark red, without sheen, and soaked in bloody oedema. The serosal coat was raised in blebs, and haemorrhage had occurred into the muscular layers. The mucosa was grossly swollen and showed a massive secretion of serosanguinous fluid. The mesenteric lymph nodes were haemorrhagic. The veins were engorged with blood but not thrombosed. These appearances are identical to those later described by Hertzler[30] and by Boyd[13] in human subjects following a mesenteric embolus. The histological appearances were those of progressive necrosis from the mucosa

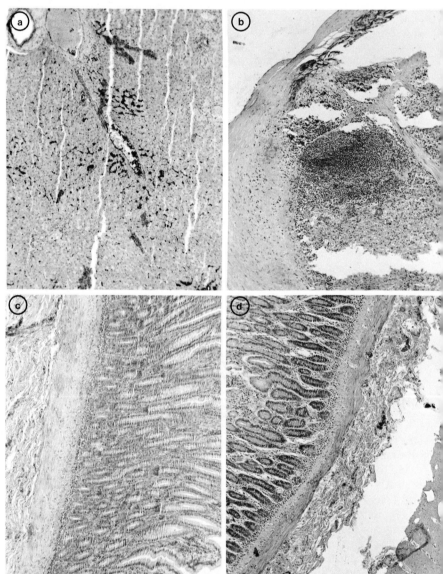

Fig. 4.1. Intra-arterial injection of graphite following SMA occlusion: (a) liver; (b) spleen; (c) terminal ileum; (d) terminal ileum following graphite injection into portal vein.

outwards, with oedema and haemorrhage; microscopy of the mesentery and bowel wall showed a backward-running venous stream and gradual filling of the veins.

The source of the haemorrhage was a matter of dispute among the early workers.

Litten clearly believed that it came from the veins. He excluded the possibility of its arriving via the arterial collateral by injecting various dyes into the left heart following SMA ligation, and demonstrating that particles were present in every tissue except the infarcted bowel. This has been confirmed since by our own group[51] (Fig. 4.1).

Welch,[85] in his studies on haemorrhagic infarction, took the opposite view and was strongly of the opinion that the haemorrhage occurred from arterial collateral to the infarct. His studies, however, were of short loops of intestine, which in the dog have an abundant arterial collateral from either end. Welch measured the arterial and venous pressures following SMA occlusion and showed that a pressure of 30 mm Hg persists in the SMA beyond the point of ligature, and a pressure of 30–50 mm Hg is recordable in the portal vein. As the SMA pressure was gradually reduced, haemorrhagic infarction occurred when it reached a value of a quarter of normal.

Later studies on the effect of SMA ligation in rats by Khanna[14, 34] confirmed the presence of an outward-spreading mucosal necrosis (which is apparent within a few minutes of ligation) and suggested that, at any rate in this animal, haemorrhage occurs from the arteries, as intraortic dye was found to enter the bowel through collaterals. No oedema and no evidence of altered capillary permeability in the serosa were observed. (The question of the origin of the haemorrhagic infarct is still disputed; there may well be species differences.)

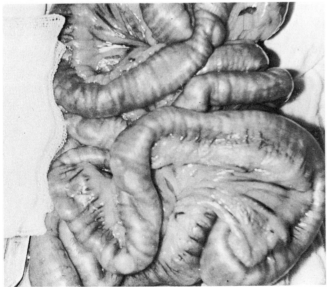

Fig. 4.2. Immediate appearances in the bowel following occlusion of the SMA.

The gross effects on the bowel are much as have been described above. The initial reaction is of spasm, with empty arteries, and the appearance of concentric pale stripes at sites of maximum ischaemia.

After 3–4 hours tone disappears and the bowel becomes cyanotic, flabby and oedematous. Over the next few hours the oedema increases, and areas of discoloration appear, most obviously at the region of the ileocaecal junction, which is that part most distant from the embryological origin of the blood supply. A sharp demarcation appears between the healthy and infarcted tissue at the duodenojejunal flexure above, and at the upper part of the descending colon below, where the superior mesenteric territory inosculates with its neighbouring great vessels. Although the bowel becomes progressively damaged and areas of greenish and even black gangrene appear, frank gangrene perforation is unusual, and in one personal series of 48 SMA ligations it was never seen.[51] Areas of quite healthy intestine may persist, and the animal usually dies before the whole of its alimentary tract has succumbed. The disappearance of peristalsis is a capricious and unreliable sign, and indeed peristalsis may be evoked in segments of bowel in an animal which has already died.

The changes in the bowel are patchy rather than uniform. This is probably due to the fact that intramural flow is sensitive to many factors, some of them mechanical, and others biochemical and hormonal. The diameter and position of an individual loop of bowel, though unimportant in the healthy individual, becomes crucial when the arterial input pressure is drastically reduced, and under these circumstances small alterations in intraluminal tension, due to areas of spasm and obstruction, may have drastic effects on intramural flow. Furthermore, the bacterial and chemical content of the bowel have been shown to have important effects on the speed of necrosis, following SMA occlusion.[11, 15, 18, 37, 64]

Two other constant features are the appearance of a moderate quality of turbid, offensive fluid in the peritoneal cavity, and the appearance of bubbles of gas in the mesenteric veins, presumably derived from bacterial activity within the lumen and wall of the gut (Fig. 4.3).

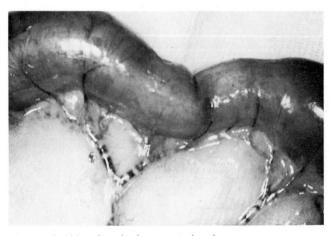

Fig. 4.3. Bubbles of gas in the mesenteric veins.

Histological appearances

The very earliest change seen following SMA occlusion is lifting of the epithelium and formation of a space (Grunhagen's space) between the glandular cells and basement membrane.[1, 16] The tips of the villi then begin to slough and a membrane of necrotic epithelium fibrin, inflammatory cells and bacteria accumulates. Later on, oedema appears, with haemorrhage

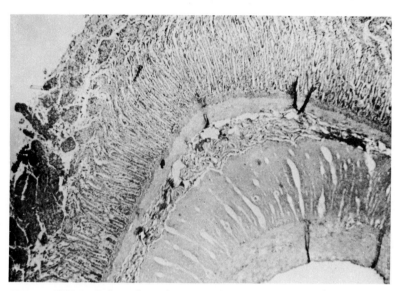

Fig. 4.4. SMA occlusion: photomicrograph of appearances at 3 hours.

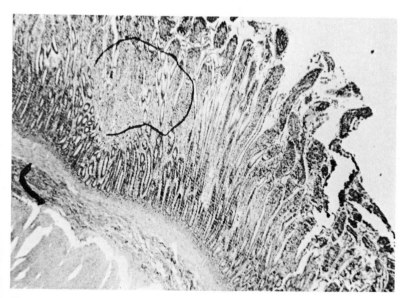

Fig. 4.5. SMA occlusion: photomicrograph of appearance at 6 hours.

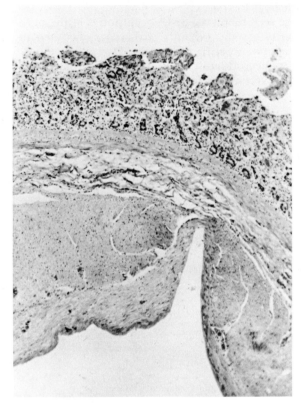

Fig. 4.6. SMA occlusion: photomicrograph of appearances at 9 hours.

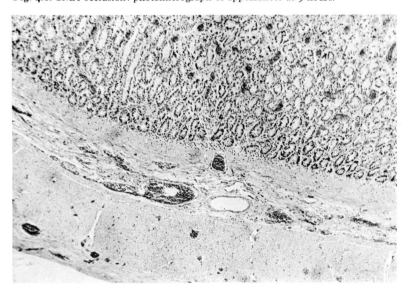

Fig. 4.7 SMA occlusion: photomicrograph to show collapsed arteries and thrombosed veins.

into the submucosa, while there is a steady progression of necrotic change from the lumen outwards until, in the worst-affected area, no trace of mucosal detail remains (see Figs. 4.4–4.6). While these events occur in the mucosa, there is progressive emptying of the arterial tree with simultaneous engorgement of the veins, some of which thrombose (see Fig. 4.7).[22, 50] The initially brisk inflammatory response in the wall of the bowel, with accumulation of polymorphonuclear leucocytes, is gradually replaced by a diminution of inflammatory cell elements, presumably due to depletion of their numbers by anoxia with no corresponding replacement from the arterial circulation. The bowel wall becomes progressively thinned as the mucosa separates and sloughs into the lumen, and at 9–10 hours (see Fig. 4.6) perforation may occur.

General effects of SMA occlusion

Gangrene of the entire midgut loop is obviously incompatible with life, and is of little clinical interest. However, a paradox exists which has been the starting point for many experimental studies. It is this: death of the individual frequently takes place before the intestine has lost all viability, and release of the experimentally occluded SMA leads to death more certainly and more quickly than if the occlusion is maintained[43, 47, 50, 55, 62, 63, 66] Total abolition of flow in the arterial side of the splanchnic circulation creates an extremely complex physiological disturbance, which is difficult to analyse, but some of the main components of this will now be discussed (Fig. 4.8).

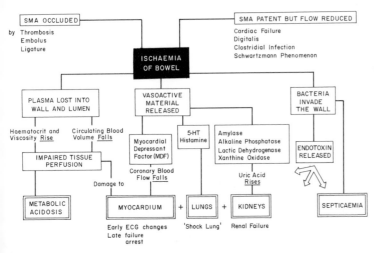

Fig. 4.8. Physiological consequences of SMA occlusion.

Redistribution of body fluid

With the realization of the importance of fluid loss in all types of intestinal obstruction,[86] interest began to centre on lethal factors in strangulation-obstruction, of which SMA occlusion may be considered a variety. Scott and Wangensteen[76] demonstrated that from 14 to 66 per cent of the blood volume was lost following strangulation of a loop of intestine, depending on the length of the loop. They assumed a putative blood volume of 7·5 per cent of body weight, and calculated losses by collecting the peritoneal exudate and weighing the bowel. Holt[31] confirmed the protective effect of saline transfusion following strangulation-obstruction. Aird,[2] with more refined techniques involving plasma dilution, measured the extent of blood loss following massive venous obstruction of the small bowel, and found this to be between 45 and 55 per cent. Death occurred in 2½ hours, and appeared to be due to haemorrhage. Taking into account the change in haematocrit, there appeared to be a selective loss of cells as against plasma (which recent studies do not confirm). It is clear nevertheless that in short-loop strangulation the main cause of death is rupture and peritonitis; in long-loop strangulation it is loss of fluid. The classical experiments aimed to reproduce the type of intestinal obstruction which is seen clinically in a strangulated hernia, so that the lesion in most cases involved a short loop of intestine, the veins, arteries and lumen of which were obstructed. This situation is rather different from total or focal ischaemia of the midgut, where the veins remain patent. But an isolated arterial lesion does, in fact, lead to gross loss of extracellular fluid.

Our group[50, 51] demonstrated in 20 dogs a mean fall in blood volume of 34 per cent between the time of SMA occlusion and death. The red cell mass during this time fell by 10 per cent while the plasma volume fell by 54 per cent on average. The haematocrit frequently reached a level of 65–70 per cent immediately before death. This massive degree of haemoconcentration and fluid loss occurred in the absence of any significant portal hypertension, so that the well known syndrome of 'hepatic outflow obstruction' which tends to occur in dogs in response to stress was ruled out as a cause. The conclusion reached on the basis of these studies was that the plasma leakage was occurring from the venous side of the circulation, into the wall and lumen of the bowel, via the damaged intestinal capillary.

These results have been confirmed recently by Tjiong,[82] who investigated the relative importance of fluid shift and metabolic change during and after occlusion of the SMA in 11 splenectomized dogs. Following measurements of blood volume and total body water the SMA was clamped; the clamp was released 4 hours later, following which the spaces were again measured, the measurement being repeated after a further 2 hours. At the same time, blood gases, serum electrolytes and osmolarity were estimated. These authors were able to confirm the major shifts in body fluids which we observed in our studies in 1962, and at the same time demonstrated that blood cultures, in spite of changes characteristic of endotoxin absorption, were negative. While blood volume, total body water, serum potassium, pCO_2 and bicarbonate all declined, the arterial pO_2 remained relatively constant.

Absorption of vasoactive material from the bowel

Vasoactive material is produced in the ischaemic bowel and absorbed via the peritoneum,[2] the veins[58] and the lymphatics.[34] Among the substances present are catecholamines,[35] histamine,[34] 5-hydroxytryptamine,[29, 61, 75] ferritin[29] and enzymes such as β-glucuronidase,[12] trans-aminase[20] and alkaline phosphatase.[74, 88] Additionally, the portal blood is hyperkalaemic[4, 58] and acidotic,[72] and is presumably rich in bacterial endotoxin.[24]

Systemic effects can be demonstrated long before gangrene, or even much tissue damage, has occurred in the ischaemic intestine.[72] Williams and his group[87] have studied early effects on the myocardium of short periods of small bowel ischaemia. Confirming and extending the earlier studies of Bounous[11] and Dogru,[23] they demonstrated that within 1 hour of occlusion of the SMA in dogs there is a substantial decrease in cardiac output, accompanied by electrocardiographic change. Examination of the peripheral blood revealed the presence of a myocardial depressant factor (MDF), identified by its effect on the isolated rat myocardial strip.[38]

Similar results were obtained by Vyden et al.,[84] who studied the cardio-vascular responses to acute occlusion of the SMA in dogs. They demon-strated initial transitory rises in arterial pressure and in coronary, renal and cerebral blood flow, which were followed by progressive increases in systemic vascular resistance with a concomitant fall off in flow to all vital organs. The observed changes occurred early, before any great change in plasma volume could have taken place, and were the opposite from what would have been expected from release of 5-HT from the damaged bowel. The authors lend their support to the view of Lefer and of Williams that a myocardial depressant factor is responsible, perhaps originating from the ischaemic pancreas.

Revascularization of the intestine

As has already been pointed out, once the SMA has been occluded for more than a few hours, release of the clamp leads to peripheral circulatory collapse and death of the animal.

The maximum tolerable period of midgut ischaemia in dogs was deter-mined by Nelson and Kremen,[63] who found that the SMA could be safely occluded for 2 hours, but that release of the ligature after 3 hours' occlusion caused death in 60 per cent of dogs, and after 4 hours' occlusion in 80 per cent. Shapiro et al.[77] found that in rabbits 1 hour's occlusion was always fatal, and that in fact death occurred more quickly if the ligature was released than if it was left in place. The result of revascularizing the ischaemic intestine was haemorrhage into the bowel, accompanied by a fall in plasma volume, and rise in haematocrit. Medins and Laufman[59] and Lillehei[40, 41, 42] found similar effects in the dog. Revascularization of the ischaemic intestine is clearly unsafe, and this may help to explain the high mortality of mesenteric embolectomy in clinical practice.

Zuidema et al.[89] found that a 2-hour period of SMA occlusion in dogs produced leakage of ^{131}I-labelled polyvinylpyrrolidone (PVP) into the bowel, lowered serum albumin, decreased fat absorption, and a transient drop in blood urea nitrogen over a period of several days. Serum sodium and potassium levels were unaffected.

We confirmed the abrupt fall in arterial blood pressure, peripheral re-sistance and blood volume which occurs following release of the occluded SMA,[49, 50, 51, 54] and demonstrated that whereas the fluid lost in the prerelease period was largely plasma, revascularization led to massive haemorrhage into the intestinal wall and lumen, in itself quite enough to account for death of the animal.

It was further shown that when a normal donor dog was cross-circulated through the ischaemic bowel, it too died, but that this death could be prevented by blood replacement, suggesting that absorption of toxic material was a less important lethal factor than was haemorrhage under these circumstances.[50]

These early studies could be challenged in that they (1) took no account of the spleen's contribution to the blood volume, (2) measured total blood volume with the use of iodinated serum albumin which is now known to be misleading, and (3) drew conclusions from cross-circulation experiments involving unmatched blood. However, later studies, using a more refined approach, have confirmed their findings. Thus Chiu et al.,[17] while admitting the importance of absorption of such toxic factors as histamine and β-glucuronidase, found that after 3 hours of SMA occlusion in splenectomized dogs the mortality could be reduced from 89 to 36 per cent by adequate fluid therapy. Flushing of the mesenteric circulation following the same period of ischaemia did not produce circulatory failure. Kangwalklai et al.[33] carried out detailed space-studies during and after 3 hours' SMA occlusion. They confirmed our findings of progressive plasma loss (actually 3·9 per cent per hour as opposed to 5 per cent per hour, but this could be accounted for by differences in experimental detail) but found much less contraction in blood and plasma volumes after release of the clamp, although there was a contraction in total, and particularly in intracellular, body water. Later figures obtained by Tjiong et al.[82] of the same research team showed greater losses of whole blood.

However, this cannot be the whole story and it is well recognized that death from revascularization of the ischaemic bowel, long before the point of necrosis is reached, is often not preventable by maintenance of a normal blood volume,[60] whereas preparation of the bowel by various measures designed to reduce endotoxin production and prevent vasoconstriction in the intestinal wall help to lower the mortality.[60, 62]

Conclusions

The controversy as regards the relative importance of fluid depletion and toxic absorption as causes of death in mesenteric vascular occlusion is still not resolved, and probably never will be. However, it does seem that provided the ischaemic damage is sufficiently slight to be wholly recoverable when the bowel is revascularized, the substances released into the systemic circulation following removal of the occlusion (potassium, histamine, 5-HT, cellular enzymes, endotoxin and vasoactive polypeptides) may not always reach concentrations high enough to cause death, provided that the circulating volume is adequately maintained.

Factors which modify the effects of SMA ligation

Factors which modify the effects of SMA ligation include the following:

Hypothermia

The tolerable period of SMA occlusion can be lengthened considerably by lowering of the body temperature,[59, 66] to the extent that if the bowel is cooled to 5°C its entire circulation can be interrupted, so that autotransplantation can be carried out.[43]

Antibiotics

Laufman[37] found that a 6-hour venous strangulation of the lower ileum in dogs was invariably fatal, whereas with massive penicillin therapy 8 out of 10 recovered, with varying degrees of stricturing and peritoneal adhesions. Rabinowici and Fine[70] produced similar results using systemic tetracycline, and Cohn[18] was able to preserve normal mucosa in completely devascularized loops of intestine, when the same drug was given into the lumen. Benjamin *et al.*[3] extended these results to show that the mortality period following SMA ligation could be extended with systemic penicillin and streptomycin.

These laboratory findings have prompted clinicians to sterilize the bowel with aminoglycoside drugs before undertaking reconstruction of the lower aorta and visceral arteries.

Similar protection from endotoxin absorption in established ischaemia can be provided by peritoneal lavage.[15]

Anticoagulants

Martin *et al.*[55] demonstrated that systemic heparin prevented sludging of blood and adherence of cells to the endothelial wall of the small gut vessels in major vascular occlusion, and this work was confirmed by Nelson and Kremen,[63] who showed a substantial reduction of mortality in SMA occlusion, and a prolongation of the safe occlusion period. The administration of low molecular weight dextran fractions[19] has also been demonstrated as useful.

α-Adrenergic blockade

Orr[65] was the first to describe the beneficial effect of splanchnic nerve block in a patient with mesenteric embolism. There has been a certain amount of confirmation of this in the experimental laboratory,[39, 60, 62] using systemically administered α-blocking agents, and regional blockade with local anaesthetics. Thus Nahor *et al.*[62] studied the effect of coeliac blockade and of intravenous and intra-aortic phenoxybenzamine on standard SMA shock in dogs and rabbits, and showed that prerelease blockade significantly lowered the death rate. When this treatment was given following restoration of blood flow, results were less good although coeliac blockade still had some effect. The exact way in which these agents improve the intestinal circulation is not clear. Any remaining arterial spasm in the intestinal wall is presumably abolished, and the collateral circulation dilated, but in circumstances of extreme anoxia the minute vessels will already have been largely paralysed. At the same time, the sympathomimetic effect of the various vasoactive polypeptides, and of bacterial endotoxin, will be counteracted. Vasodilatation in the liver and spleen may also be of importance. There is, furthermore, some evidence that α-adrenergic blockade is capable of preventing the myocardial lesion which occurs in experimental endotoxin shock.[90]

Abolition of tryptic activity

Gurd and his associates at McGill University have drawn attention to the importance of conditions within the intestinal lumen in the development of haemorrhagic lesions in the intestine in low-output states, or in experimentally induced ischaemia. An important cause of death in canine shock is intestinal autolysis associated with tryptic activity. Their work[11] has demonstrated that a 90-minute occlusion period of both SMA and IMA produces demonstrable lesions in the heart and kidney, which can be prevented by preoperative feeding of an elemental diet. The diet consists of amino acids, sucrose, electrolytes and vitamins, and when the standard ischaemic challenge is given the extraintestinal lesions fail to appear. It appears that pancreatic proteolytic enzymes present in the lumen of the bowel are involved in the pathogenesis of the haemorrhagic intestinal necrosis, and that such enzymic activity can be abolished by altering the intraluminal content.

However, Manohar[47] has found that ligation of the pancreatic duct, which abolished tryptic enteritis, does not in fact lessen the mortality from SMA shock, and that sterilization of the bowel has little effect. Survival time is prolonged by intravenous fluid therapy and cortisol.

Intraluminal oxygen

Haglund[27, 28] found that small amounts of oxygen supplied to the mucosa via an intraluminal perfusion of oxygenated saline could prevent the development of haemorrhagic lesions in the tips of the villi, which occur during periods of reduced intestinal blood flow. This effect was not seen when nitrogenated saline was used.

This work has been extended by Shute[78] who found an 89 per cent mortality and gross histological damage to the bowel in rats subjected to SMA occlusion for 2 hours, which could be reduced to 29 per cent (with correspondingly reduced damage) by the use of gaseous oxygen introduced into the lumen. He suggests possible clinical application of these results.

Chronic occlusion of the SMA and other main arteries

Gradual obliteration of the SMA is not lethal to man, but may lead to disease. Recognition of this has led to many laboratory studies, the first of which was by Blalock and Levy[6] whose interest, in fact, was not in intestinal ischaemia *per se*, but in the regulation of the arterial blood pressure. Following Goldblatt's demonstration that constriction of the renal artery gave rise to hypertension, they sought for this property in various other vessels, with negative results. By selective constriction of the coeliac axis, SMA and IMA with Goldblatt clamps, Blalock and Levy were able to obtain 7 surviving dogs out of 29 whose intestinal arteries were completely closed. These animals appeared to be in good health, and no gross abnormalities were found post mortem. Detailed studies of the bowel were not done.

Laufman[36] obtained complete occlusion of the SMA in 2 out of 5 dogs over a period of 4 months, by wrapping Cellophane tape around the origin of the vessel. These animals suffered a severe systemic upset, lost weight and became anaemic. Some pallor of the bowel and mucosal destruction was noted. Later, Spencer and Derrick[79] reported on a series of 7 dogs in which they narrowed the SMA to an estimated 66–91 per cent of its original diameter with a thread ligature. These animals again showed weight loss, diarrhoea and epilation over a 4-month period, at the end of which they were sacrificed. A control dog in whom the same dissection was performed, but the ligature left loose, remained in good health. Pallor of the bowel was noted post mortem.

In none of these three series of experiments were detailed biochemical, radiological or histological observations made. Chronic midgut ischaemia was not investigated fully in the laboratory, until we restudied the problem in 1964[51] using the Ameroid cylinder technique. (Ameroid is a plastic which has the property of expanding at a constant rate when it is wet, so that, if outward expansion is prevented, any structure enclosed within it will be predictably compressed.[5]) Fourteen dogs were used in these experiments. Following a baseline estimation of weight, haematocrit serum levels of B_{12} and folate, and a d-xylose absorption test, the collateral circulation above and below the superior mesenteric arterial territory was divided, and an Ameroid cylinder positioned around the origin of the SMA. It was calculated that obliteration of the lumen of the vessel would be complete at about 3 weeks, and this was confirmed by aortography and a subsequent laparotomy, at which the bowel was biopsied (Fig. 4.9).

Apart from a transient disturbance some 4–7 days after insertion of the Ameroid, no obvious clinical abnormality was noticed in these dogs. At the final laparotomy, the bowel appeared pale but otherwise normal, and no pulsations could be detected in the arcades. A pressure gradient of 100 mm Hg was generally found across the occluded segment of artery. Vascular adhesions had formed around the Ameroid, the loops of bowel and the abdominal incisions.[25] There appeared to be no hypertrophy of the coeliac axis, inferior mesenteric artery, or lumbar and lower intercostal branches, and aortography (Fig. 4.9b) showed that the bowel was nourished by a network of fine collaterals originating from extracoelomic vessels. No specific abnormalities were found in the serum folate and B_{12} level although there was some drop in haematocrit. The xylose absorption studies were not conclusive and probably reflected the inaccuracy of the method (Fig. 4.10). Over all, absorption tended to decrease over the first 6 weeks and then gradually to revert to normal. There was little correlation between xylose excretion, haematocrit, and body weight, which often tended to shift independently. Biopsies of the lower ileum obtained at intervals of from 3 to 13 weeks postoperatively were completely normal.[51]

Similar studies using an Ameroid cylinder were carried out by Popovsky.[69] These, too, had negative results.

In other words, the early results of Laufmann, and of Spencer and Derrick, could not be repeated.

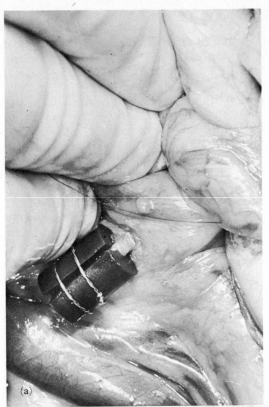

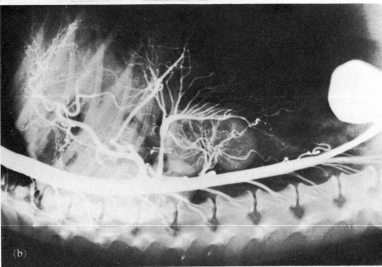

Fig. 4.9. Chronic occlusion of SMA: (a) the Ameroid cylinder in position; (b) angiogram to demonstrate collateral circulation. (Note post-stenotic dilatation of SMA and enlargement of branches of IMA.)

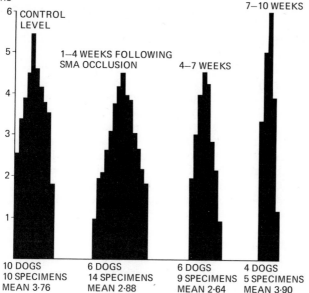

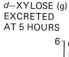

Fig. 4.10. *d*-Xylose absorption in 10 dogs following chronic occlusion of SMA. (Reproduced from Marston, *Annals of the Royal College of Surgeons of England*, 1964, **35**: 175, by kind permission of the Honorary Editor.)

Although it is possible to produce chronic obliteration of the mesenteric arteries in the experimental laboratory, the lesions do not correlate with intestinal function.

Occlusion of segmental vessels

The small intestine

It is less easy than might be thought to produce consistent lesions in the small intestine by interference with the regional blood supply. Such attempts usually either kill the animal from intestinal rupture and peritonitis, or else have no demonstrable effect on the bowel. Litten[44] ligated jejunal and ileal arteries in 19 dogs, and found no intestinal damage. Maass[45] was able to demonstrate stenosis of the small intestine in rabbits, after temporary interruption of the blood supply, but most later studies[9, 10, 83] have not succeeded in causing parenchymal lesions unless both arteries and veins have been interrupted.

Glotzer[26] constructed an isolated jejunal loop in 17 dogs, and at a second operation produced mucosal ischaemia by constricting the pedicle of the loop for between 2 and 8 hours. Eight-hour periods of ischaemia resulted in gangrene of the loop and death of the animal. The depth of damage in the other groups was directly proportional to the duration of ischaemia, as was the period necessary for healing, which was between 1 and 100 days.

The significance of this study was that it showed that complete repair, not only of the mucosa but of the smooth muscle in the villi, was possible after even a very deep ischaemic injury. Additionally, the regenerated villi were seen to be short, irregular, thick and branching, resembling the appearances found in coeliac disease, or following radiation injury (see also Chapter 7).

Our experience[51] was disappointing, in that ligation of the arcade vessels produced neither gross nor histological abnormality. The same findings were obtained by Vest and Margulis,[83] who showed that interruption of these vessels resulted either in no change at all or in gangrene, perforation and death. There are, as already mentioned, significant differences between the vascular architecture of different species, and this may well account for the discrepancies between the results. None the less, it is recognized that an ischaemic insult which is not sufficiently prolonged or severe to lead to gangrene, but at the same time prevents normal regeneration of the specialized layers of the bowel, can produce lasting damage, usually in the form of a fibrous stricture[61, 81] (see also Chapter 7).

The 'potassium stricture'

A particular form of ischaemic damage in the small intestine is that caused by the application of high concentrations of potassium ion to the mucosa. This has particular relevance to the strictures encountered clinically in association with enteric-coated potassium chloride tablets. Stahlgren[80] demonstrated that potassium chloride, alone or in combination with thiazide diuretics, could produce focal mucosal ulceration, which sometimes progressed to fibrosis and stricture formation. This was particularly prone to occur if the arterial arcades to the segment had been divided which in itself, as already explained, is not a damaging situation in the small intestine. The fact that pre-existing intestinal ischaemia is particularly likely to give rise to potassium stricture was underlined by the work of Mansfield,[46] who showed that animals with an experimentally constructed pressure gradient across the SMA were particularly vulnerable to insult by potassium. They pointed out that ulceration took place at the site of lymphoid follicles, which tallies with the clinical observation that most of these lesions occur in the ileum, where lymphoid tissue is concentrated. This is discussed further in Chapter 7.

The colon

The original experiments on acute segmental colonic ischaemia were carried out by Hukuhara *et al.*[32] in 1961. These authors were interested in the causation of congenital megacolon, and in 4 dogs produced a 4-hour ischaemia period by isolating a segment of colon on a vascular pedicle perfused with Tyrode solution. They carried out barium studies at intervals in the postoperative period, and eventually sacrificed the animals for histological examination. They demonstrated contraction of the gut in a region corresponding to the perfused segment, but this area could be distended by increasing the head of pressure by barium, and the authors concluded that the stricture was of a functional rather than a structural nature. Pathological appearances showed contracture and shortening of the bowel, but no mucosal ulceration. Histological abnormalities were comparatively minor, but no normal ganglion cells were found in the myoepithelial plexuses.

It is interesting that later work by de Villiers,[21] using an almost identical technique, produced contrasting results in that there were marked changes in the mucosa and muscle layers of the ischaemic segments, but ganglion cells were present in every specimen examined. De Villiers completely failed to reproduce the results of the Japanese workers, and could not concur in postulating ischaemia as a possible factor in the genesis of congenital aganglionosis.

Further studies in experimental devascularization of the colon were carried out by Boley and his group.[7] These authors were interested in the clinical and radiological aspects of colonic ischaemia, and were able to reproduce in the laboratory their clinical experience, by ligating the dog's intestinal arteries at or distal to the arcades. They followed up these studies[8] by a further series of experiments in which glass and ceramic microspheres of known diameter were injected into the caudal mesenteric artery via the aorta. They noted blanching and contraction of the involved segment during the injection, which usually disappeared when the arterial clamps were released and blood flow was resumed. If the colour of the bowel did not return to normal, necrosis followed (although, conversely, return of normal colour did not preclude subsequent necrosis). According to the size and quantity of the microspheres injected, a varying degree of streaking, superficial ulceration, inflammation, perforation and eventual stricture formation was observed. Barium enemas were carried out under anaesthesia and showed 'thumb-printing', ulceration and late stenosis. No histological studies were reported by these authors.

Studies in our laboratory[52] confirmed and extended this work. In these experiments standardized vascular interruptions were carried out as follows (Fig. 4.11):

1. Ligation of the caudal mesenteric artery.
2. Ligation of the caudal mesenteric artery and marginal artery.
3. Ligation of the caudal mesenteric and marginal arteries, plus the common colic artery.

Following operation, the animals were sacrificed at 1, 14 and 42 days. Observations made during the experimental period included routine clinical examination, sigmoidoscopy, barium enema, leucocyte count, and estimation of alkaline phosphatase, lactic dehydrogenase, aspartate transaminase and glutamate transaminase. In addition, all the lesions were examined both grossly and microscopically.

The aim of these studies was to reproduce as far as possible the effects of a mesenteric thrombosis affecting the colon. For this reason it was considered better simply to ligate the vessels, rather than to introduce the added factors of intravascular foreign bodies or of the gross alterations in tissue electrolyte concentrations which are bound to occur following perfusion with saline or Tyrode solution. By varying the site of vascular interruption and by studying the lesions at successive degrees of maturity,

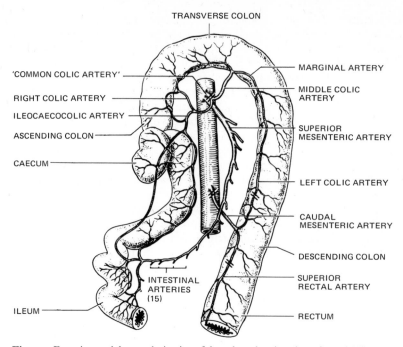

Fig. 4.11 Experimental devascularization of the colon, showing sites of arterial ligation (Reproduced from Marston *et al.*, *Gut*, 1969, **10**: 24, by kind permission of the Editor.)

it was hoped to obtain some information regarding the natural history of the condition. The main findings of this study were as follows.

Ligation of the caudal mesenteric artery alone has little effect, but even quite severe degrees of colonic ischaemia are well tolerated by the healthy animal and do not usually cause a major systemic illness.

The most striking changes seen on *sigmoidoscopy* occurred the day following the operation, and consisted in a circumferential mucosal slough at the recto-sigmoid junction with intense congestion above and below (Fig. 4.12). At 14 days small discrete ulcers were seen and at 6 weeks these were followed by stricture formation and contact bleeding. Less florid lesions, such as spasm, mucosal oedema, and haemorrhage into the submucous lymphoid follicles, were frequent. Ligation of the caudal mesenteric artery alone produced minor abnormalities in 1 animal out of 6, the remaining 5 being unaffected.

The earliest *radiological change* was 'thumb-printing' of the affected segment, due to spasm, mucosal oedema and haemorrhage, which usually reverted to normal within a few weeks although occasionally a persistent stenosis resulted. The ulceration which was seen through the sigmoidoscope and on the pathological specimens proved difficult to demonstrate radiologically (Fig. 4.13).

Histopathological changes varied from surface inflammation to heavy deposition of fibrous tissue, depending on the extent and maturity of the lesion (Fig. 4.14). A conspicuous feature was the presence of haemosiderin-laden macrophages in the submucosa (see also Chapter 9).

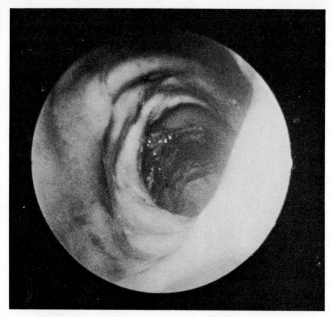

Fig. 4.12. Sigmoidoscopic appearance 2 weeks following ligation of the caudal mesenteric artery (CMA) and the marginal artery (MA)—a circumferential slough has developed.

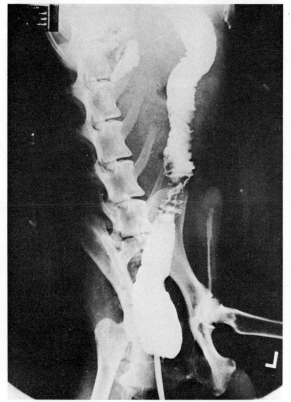

Fig. 4.13. Barium enema 42 days following ligation of the caudal mesenteric artery (CMA) and the marginal artery (MA), showing: above, early change—'thumb-printing'; and, below, late change—stricture.

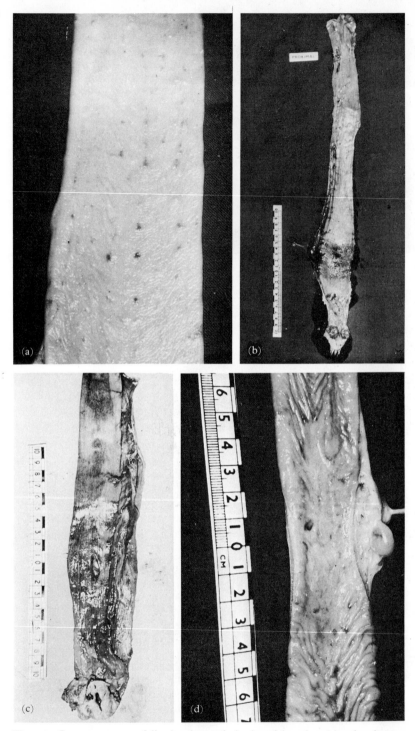

Fig. 4.14. Gross appearances following devascularization of the colon: (a) early minor vascular injury; (b and c) early major vascular injury; (d) late changes, showing stricture formation.

There was a sharp rise in circulating leucocytes following the operation in all cases, which seemed unrelated to the degree of vascular injury.

Postoperative levels of lactic dehydrogenase and of aspartate and glutamate transaminases did not vary significantly from the preoperative baseline. However, the serum level of alkaline phosphatase rose abruptly in the immediate postoperative period, and this rise was directly related to the extent of devascularization and mucosal necrosis (Fig. 4.15). This finding prompted the question as to whether intestinal isoenzyme was being released into the circulation by the damaged bowel, which might form the basis of a potentially useful laboratory test for acute intestinal ischaemia.[74] However, when the isoenzymes were separated, no preponderance was found of the intestinal fraction, and the observed rise in alkaline phosphatase appeared to be coming from the liver. The differences noted between the groups of major colonic injury and the controls suggested, however, that the rise in enzyme level is not purely the result of handling of the liver during the operation because this happens to the same extent in both groups. A possible explanation is that the damaged colon leads to portal bacteraemia, which provokes an outpouring of the hepatic enzyme. However, without bacteriological examination of the portal blood, this must remain a speculation.

Further studies from our laboratory[48] were concerned with venous lesions of the colon. Initially, attempts were made to produce thrombosis of the inferior mesenteric vein by the simple application of ligatures, but those were unsuccessful. Subsequently, an isolated segment of vein was thrombosed by injecting thrombin according to the technique originally described by Polk.[68] In 13 dogs so treated, severe lesions were produced.

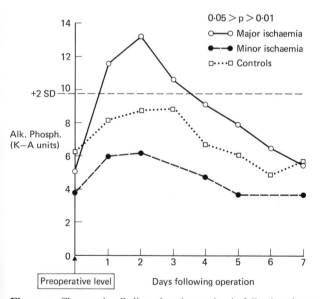

Fig. 4.15. Changes in alkaline phosphatase levels following devascularization of the colon, in relation to the degree of vascular injury. (Reproduced from Marston *et al.*, *Gut*, 1969, **10**: 24, by kind permission of the Editor.)

There were some notable differences between the arterial and the venous occlusions. In the acute stages both showed congestion and oedema of the submucosa, but mucosal necrosis, which is so frequent in arterial lesions, was not found in those caused by interference with the veins. When it occurs, venous gangrene appears to affect mainly the submucosa and is usually associated with total necrosis of the muscle; the mucosa may be lost as a secondary process. The early histological picture shows congestion and dilatation of lymphatics and collateral veins. In the later stages, after resolution, there was evidence of erythrocyte sequestration, as seen by deposition of haemosiderin in the submucosa, and also in the regional mesenteric lymph nodes, the latter feature being highly characteristic. Sigmoidoscopy revealed widespread blue congestion of the mucosa, as distinct from the pale slough which appears following arterial interruption. The radiological and sigmoidoscopic features correlated well, particularly in the more severe cases, and 'thumb-printing' was more obvious after venous thrombosis. The changes in leucocyte count and serum enzyme levels following venous interruption were much the same as had been seen with arterial lesions.

The group of workers from Lausanne[71, 73] has for some years been interested in the functional as well as the morphological response of the colon to ischaemia. They have used a technique of total colonic ischaemia induced by clamping all afferent arteries for different periods of time, following which measurements of sodium flux, together with concentrations of Na/K/ATPase, across the mucosa, are measured. The morphological changes produced were very much as have been described above.[52] The authors draw attention to the comparatively slight effects of short ischaemic periods on the colonic mucosa, contrasting to the autolytic destruction seen in the ileum after similar challenge. In this study two groups of dogs were used: an acute group in which the colons were removed for functional studies, and a recovery group in which the maturation of the lesion could be studied and its function estimated weeks later. It was found that active sodium transport disappeared after 2 hours of ischaemia, although ATPase activity persisted. Sodium flux was not a very convenient or reliable determinant of colonic function in the more severe lesions but Na/K/ATPase levels correlated well with recoverability, and the authors suggest that it may prove to be a useful clinical test. Matthews and Parks[57] have confirmed these results and have shown that when SMA flow is reduced to below 20 per cent of normal, absorption of sodium ion is replaced by net secretion. They suggest that this may help to explain the diarrhoea observed in chronic intestinal ischaemia, in that the diarrhoea may originate in the small bowel and that the ischaemic colon, being unable to absorb the fluid bulk, acts as a passive tube for the transport of unaltered ileal contents.[57]

These same workers[56, 67] have made the extremely interesting observation that gradual occlusion of common colic and caudal mesenteric arteries in the dog does not bring about functional change in the colon, but that when SMA flow in such an animal is abruptly lowered by hypotensive drugs or venesection, then ischaemic changes in the colon are precipitated. This goes far to explain how ischaemic colitis can occur acutely in the clinical situation, without there being an acute occlusion of a colonic blood vessel.

Conclusions

In contrast to what obtains in the small intestine, experimental interference with the regional circulation to the colon is capable of producing predictable lesions, in both the short and the long term. Functional impairment may occur before there is any discernible anatomical change. Ischaemia produces transient superficial inflammation, linear ulceration progressing to loss of mucosa, fulminating inflammation and full-thickness necrosis, according to its degree and duration. Later lesions include chronic ulceration, and strictures of the colon due to the deposition of fibrous tissue in the submucosa. Broadly speaking, the morphological changes found following deliberate devascularization of the colon in the experimental animal are similar to those seen in human patients suffering from ischaemic colitis, bearing in mind that the very early changes created and studied in the experimental laboratory do not often come the way of the clinical pathologist, who is usually presented with a mature and florid lesion.

References

1 Ahren, C. and Haglund, U. (1973). Mucosal lesions in the small intestine of the cat during low flow. *Acta Physiologica Scandinavica* **88**: 1–9.

2 Aird, I. (1941). Strangulation obstruction. *Annals of Surgery* **114**: 385–397.

3 Benjamin, H. B., Potos, W. B., Marnocha, J. and Bartenbach, G. E. (1960). Correlation of clinical and experimental effects of antibiotic therapy for massive intestinal infarction secondary to acute mesenteric vascular occlusion. *Journal of the American Geriatrics Society* **8**: 847–854.

4 Bergan, J. J., Gilliland, V., Troop, C. and Anderson, M. C. (1964). Hyperkalaemia following intestinal revascularization. *Journal of the American Medical Association* **187**: 17–21.

5 Berman, J. K., Fields, D. C., Judy, H., Mori, V. and Parker, R. J. (1956). The technique of gradual occlusion of large arteries using Ameroid cylinders. *Surgery* **39**: 399.

6 Blalock, A. and Levy, S. E. (1939). Gradual complete occlusion of the celiac axis and superior and inferior mesenteric arteries with survival. *Surgery* **5**: 175–180.

7 Boley, S. J., Schwartz, S., Lash, J. and Sternhill, V. (1963). Reversible vascular occlusion of the colon. *Surgery, Gynecology and Obstetrics* **116**: 53–60.

8 Boley, S. J., Krieger, H., Schultz, L., Robinson, K., Siew, F. P., Allen, A. C. and Schwartz, S. (1965). Experimental aspects of peripheral vascular occlusion of the intestine. *Surgery, Gynecology and Obstetrics* **121**: 789–794.

9 Bolognesi, G. (1909) D l'occlusion expérimentale des vaisseaux mesenteriques. *Zentralblatt für Chirurgie* **36**: 1641–1647.

10 Bonakdarpour, A., Ming, S., Lynch, P. R., Essa, N. and Reichle, F. (1975) Superior mesenteric artery occlusion in dogs: a model to produce the spectrum of intestinal ischemia. *Journal of Surgical Research* **19**: 251–257.

11 Bounous, G., Brown, R., Mulder, D. S., Hampson, L. G. and Gurd, F. N. (1965). Abolition of tryptic enteritis in the shocked dog. *Archives of Surgery* **91**: 371–376.

12 Bounous, G. and McArdle, A. H. (1969). Release of intestinal enzymes in acute ischaemia. *Journal of Surgical Research* **9**: 339–345.

13 Boyd, W. (1947). *Surgical Pathology*, 6th edn., Philadelphia, Pa., and Eastbourne, W. B. Saunders Co. p. 565.

14 Cameron, G. R. and Khanna, S. D. (1959). Regeneration of intestinal villi after extensive mucosal infarction. *Journal of Pathology and Bacteriology* **77**: 505–509.

15 Caridis, D. T., Cuevas, P. and Fine, J. (1972). Treatment of acute ischemia of the intestine by peritoneal lavage in the rabbit. *Surgery, Gynecology and Obstetrics* **135**: 199–202.

16 Chiu, C. J., McArdle, A. H., Brown, R. and Scott, H. J. (1970). Intestinal mucosal lesion in low-flow states. *Archives of Surgery* **101**: 478–483.

17 Chiu, C. J., Scott, H. J. and Gurd, F. N. (1972). Volume deficit versus toxic absorption—a study of canine shock after mesenteric arterial occlusion. *Annals of Surgery* **175**: 479–488.

18 Cohn, I. (1956). Strangulation obstruction. *Surgery* **39**: 630–634.

19 D'Angelo, G. J., Ameriso, L. M. and Tredway, J. B. (1963). Survival after mesenteric vascular occlusion by treatment with low-molecular weight dextran. *Circulation Research* **27**: 662–663.

20 Dagher, F. J., Panossian, A. and Saab, S. (1967). The effect of experimental ligation of the superior mesenteric artery on serum xanthine oxidase activity and transaminase activity. *Surgery* **62**: 1044–1050.

21 de Villiers, D. R. (1966). Ischaemia of the colon. An experimental study. *British Journal of Surgery* **53**: 497–503.

22 Devin, R. (1974). Physiopathologie de l'infarctus entéro-mésentérique. In: *Chirurgie des Arteriopathies Digestives*, pp. 225–232. Paris, Expansion Scientifique Française.

23 Dogru, M. and Atasoy, H. (1967). La répercussion de l'Ischémie gastrointestinale aigüe sur le cœur. *Bulletin de la Société Internationale de Chirurgie* **26**: 536–545.

24 Einheber, A. (1961). Proceedings of a Conference on Recent Progress and Present Problems in the Field of Shock. *Federation Proceedings*, Suppl. No. 9, p. 170. Washington, DC, Federation of The American Society of Experimental Biology.

25 Ellis, H. (1962). The aetiology of post-operative adhesions. *Proceedings of the Royal Society of Medicine* **55**: 599–600.

26 Glotzer, D. J., Villegas, A. H., Anekayama, S. and Shaw, R. S. (1962). Healing of the intestine in experimental bowel infarction. *Annals of Surgery* **155**: 183–189.

27 Haglund, U. (1973). The small intestine in hypotension and haemorrhage. *Acta Physiologica Scandinavica*, Suppl. 387, 1–37.

28 Haglund, U. and Lundgren, O. (1974). The small intestine in haemorrhagic shock. *Gastroenterology* **66**: 625–627.

29 Hershey, S. G., Baez, S. and Rovenstine, E. A. (1960). Intestinal ischemic shock in normal and dibenzyline protected dogs. *American Journal of Physiology* **200**: 1239–1245.

30 Hertler, A. E. (1935). *Surgical Pathology of the Peritoneum*. Philadelphia, Pa., J. B. Lippincott.

31 Holt, R. L. (1934). The pathology of acute strangulation of the intestine. *British Journal of Surgery* **21**: 582–587.

32 Hukuhara, T., Kotani, S. and Sato, G. (1961). Effects of destruction of intramural ganglion cells on colon motility: possible genesis of congenital megacolon. *Japanese Journal of Physiology* **11**: 635–640.

33 Kangwalklai, K., Saadat, S., Bella, E. and Enquist, I. F. (1973) Space studies

during occlusions of the superior mesenteric artery and upon its release. *Surgery, Gynecology and Obstetrics* **137**: 263–266.

34 Khanna, S. D. (1959). An experimental study of mesenteric occlusion. *Journal of Pathology and Bacteriology* **77**: 575–581.

35 Kobold, E. E. and Thal, A. P. (1963). Quantitation and identification of vaso-active substances liberated during various types of experimental intestinal ischemia. *Surgery, Gynecology and Obstetrics* **117**: 315–322.

36 Laufman, H. (1943). Gradual occlusion of the mesenteric vessels—an experimental study. *Surgery* **13**: 406–411.

37 Laufman, H. (1950). Experimental evidence of factors concerned in the eventual recovery of strangulated intestine—the effects of massive penicillin therapy. *Surgery* **28**: 509–513.

38 Lefer, A. M. (1970). Role of a myocardial depressant factor in the pathogenesis of hæmorrhagic shock. *Federation Proceedings* **29**: 1836–1840.

39 Liang, H., Bernard, H. R. and Dodd, R. B. (1961). The effect of epidural block on experimental mesenteric occlusion. *Archives of Surgery* **83**: 409–412.

40 Lillehei, R. C. (1956). The prevention of irreversible hemorrhagic shock in dogs by controlled cross-perfusion of the superior mesenteric artery. *Surgical Forum* **7**: 6–11.

41 Lillehei, R. C. (1957). The intestinal factor in irreversible hemorrhagic shock. *Surgery* **42**: 1043–1050.

42 Lillehei, R. C. and Maclean, L. D. (1958). The intestinal factor in irreversible endotoxin shock. *Annals of Surgery* **148**: 513–517.

43 Lillehei, R. C., Goott, B. and Miller, F. A. (1959). The physiological response of the small bowel of the dog to ischemia, including prolonged in vitro preservation of the bowel in successful replacement and survival. *Annals of Surgery* **150**: 543–560.

44 Litten, M. (1875). Uber die Folgen des Verschlusses der Arteria meseraica superior. *Virchows Archiv für Pathologische Anatomie* **63**: 289–312.

45 Maass, V. (1895). Uber die Entstahung von Darmenstenose nach Brucheinklemmung. *Deutsche Medizinische Wochenschrift* **21**: 365–367.

46 Mansfield, J. B., Schoenfeld, F. B., Suwa, M., Geurkink, R. E. and Anderson, M. C. (1967). The role of vascular insufficiency in drug induced small bowel ulceration. *American Journal of Surgery* **113**: 608–614.

47 Manohar, M. and Tyagi, R. (1973). Experimental intestinal ischemia shock in dogs. *American Journal of Physiology* **225**: 887–892.

48 Marcuson, R. W., Stewart, J. O. and Marston, A. (1972). Experimental venous lesions of the colon. *Gut* **13**: 1–7.

49 Marston, A., McCombs, L. and Lundquist, E. (1962). Unpublished observations.

50 Marston, A. (1963). Causes of death in mesenteric arterial occlusion. *Annals of Surgery* **158**: 952–960.

51 Marston, A. (1964). Patterns of intestinal ischaemia. *Annals of the Royal College of Surgeons of England* **35**: 151–181.

52 Marston, A., Marcuson, R. W., Chapman, M. and Arthur, J. F. (1969). Experimental study of devascularization of the colon. *Gut* **10**: 121–130.

53 Marston, A. (1972). Basic structure and function of the intestinal circulation. *Clinics in Gastroenterology* **1**: 539–546.

54 Marston, A. (1972). Diagnosis and management of intestinal ischaemia. *Annals of the Royal College of Surgeons* **50**: 29–44.

55 Martin, W. B., Laufman, H. and Tuell, S. W. (1949). Rationale of therapy in acute vascular occlusions based on micrometric observations. *Annals of Surgery* **129**: 476–481.

56   Matthews, J. G. W. and Parks, T. G. (1972). Production of ischaemic colitis experimentally in the dog by vasoconstriction and hypotensive techniques. *Gut* **13**: 323.

57   Matthews, J. G. W. and Parks, T. G. (1976). Ischaemic colitis in the experimental animal: I. Comparison of the effects of acute and subacute vascular occlusion; II. Role of hypovolaemia in the production of the disease. *Gut* **17**: 671–677.

58   Mavor, G. E., Layall, A. D., Chrystal, K. M. R. and Proctor, D. M. (1963). Mesenteric infarction as a vasocular emergency. *British Journal of Surgery* **50**: 536–539.

59   Medins, G. and Laufman, H. (1958). Hypothermia in mesenteric arterial and venous occlusion. *Annals of Surgery* **148**: 740–751.

60   Milliken, J., Nahor, A. and Fine, J. (1965). A study of the factors involved in the development of peripheral vascular collapse following release of the occluded superior mesenteric artery. *British Journal of Surgery* **52**: 699–703.

61   Mustala, O., Alfthan, O. and Peltokallio, P. (1968). 5-Hydroxytryptamine concentration of the total blood of rabbits following occlusion of the superior mesenteric artery. *Acta Chirurgica Scandinavica* **134**: 275–279.

62   Nahor, A., Milliken, J. and Fine, J. (1966). Effect of celiac blockade and dibenzyline on traumatic shock following release of occluded superior mesenteric artery. *Annals of Surgery* **163**: 29–34.

63   Nelson, L. E. and Kremen, A. J. (1950). Experimental occlusion of the superior mesenteric vessels with special reference to the role of intravascular thrombosis and its prevention by heparin and sulphasuxidine. *Surgery* **28**: 819–824.

64   Noonan, C. D., Rambo, O. N. and Margulis, A. R. (1968). Effect of timed occlusion at various levels of mesenteric arteries and veins. *Radiology* **90**, 99–106.

65   Orr, T. G., Lorhan, P. H. and Kaul, P. G. (1954). Mesenteric vascular occlusion—report of 2 cases. *Journal of the American Medical Association* **155**: 648–651.

66   Parkins, W. H., Ben, M. and Vars, H. M. (1955). Tolerance of temporary occlusion of the thoracic aorta in normothermic and hypothermic dogs. *Surgery* **38**: 38–43.

67   Parks, T. G. (1974). Experimental non-gangrenous mesenteric ischaemia. *Acta Gastroenterologica Belgica* **37**: 529–538.

68   Polk, H. C. (1966). Experimental mesenteric venous occlusion. III. Diagnosis and treatment of induced mesenteric venous thrombosis. *Annals of Surgery* **163**: 432–444.

69   Popovsky, J. (1966). Gradual occlusion of mesenteric vessels with Ameroid clamp. *Archives of Surgery* **92**: 202–205.

70   Rabinowici, N. and Fine, J. (1951). Effect of aureomycin on revascularization of dog's intestine. *Journal of Mount Sinai Hospital* **18**: 90–94.

71   Rausis, C., Robinson, J. W. I., Mirkovitch, V. and Saegesser, F. (1972). Perspectives expérimentales et cliniques dans l'insuffisance vasculaire du gros intestin. *Journal de Chirurgie* **104**: 569–576.

72   Robertson, G., Lyall, A. and Macrae, J. G. C. (1969). Acid base disturbances in mesenteric occlusion. *Surgery, Gynecology and Obstetrics* **128**: 15–20.

73   Robinson, J. W. L., Rausis, C., Basset, P. and Mirkovitch, V. (1972). Functional and morphological response of the dog colon to ischaemia. *Gut* **13**: 775–783.

74   Rosato, F. E., Lazitin, L., Miller, L. D. and Tsou, K. C. (1971). Changes in intestinal alkaline phosphatase in bowel ischemia. *American Journal of Surgery* **121**: 289–292.

75   Rosenberg, J. C. (1964). Circulating serotonin and catecholamines following occlusion of the superior mesenteric artery. *Annals of Surgery* **160**: 1062–1065.

76 Scott, H. G. and Wangensteen, O. H. (1932). Blood losses in experimental intestinal strangulations. *Proceedings of the Society for Experimental Biology and Medicine* **29**: 748–752.

77 Shapiro, P. B., Bronsther, B., Frank, E. D. and Fine, J. (1958). Host resistance to hemorrhagic shock. *Proceedings of the Society for Experimental Biology and Medicine* **97**: 372.

78 Shute, K. (1977). The effect of intraluminal oxygen on experimental acute ischaemia of the intestine. *Gut*. In the Press.

79 Spencer, D. C. and Derrick, J. R. (1962). Acute and chronic effects of constricting the superior mesenteric artery in the experimental animal. *American Surgeon* **28**: 170–173.

80 Stahlgren, L. H., Dapena, A. and Roy, R. L. (1965). Ulcerogenic properties of enteric coated compounds in dogs. *Surgical Forum* **16**: 367–370.

81 Stipa, S., Brondi, C., Cavallaro, A. and Tafuri, S. (1967). Ricerche sperimentali sulla ischemia acuta intestinale. *Bulletin de la Societé Internationale de Chirurgie* **26**: 521–535.

82 Tjiong, B., Bella, E., Weiner, M. and Enquist, I. F. (1974). Fluid shifts and metabolic changes during and after occlusion of the S.M.A. *Surgery, Gynecology and Obstetrics* **139**: 217–221.

83 Vest, B. and Margulis, A. R. (1964). Experimental infarction of the small bowel in dogs. *American Journal of Roentgenology* **92**: 1080–1087.

84 Vyden, J. K., Nagasawa, K. and Corday, E. (1974). Hemodynamic consequences of acute occlusion of the superior mesenteric artery. *American Journal of Cardiology* **34**: 687–690.

85 Welch, W. H. (1920). *Haemorrhagic Infarction. Collected Papers*, Vol. 1, pp. 66–109.

86 Wilkie, D. P. D. (1931). Experimental observations on the cause of death in acute intestinal obstruction. *British Medical Journal* **2**: 1064.

87 Williams, L. F., Goldberg, A. H., Polansky, B. J. and Byrne, J. J. (1969). Myocardial effects of intestinal ischemia. *Journal of Surgical Research* **9**: 319–322.

88 Zimmerman, H. J. and West, M. (1964). Serum enzyme changes in intestinal ischemia. *Medical Clinics of North America* **48**: 189–195.

89 Zuidema, G. D., Turcote, J. G., Wolfman, E. F. and Child, C. G. (1962). Metabolic studies in acite small bowel ischemia. *Archives of Surgery* **85**: 103–135.

90 Zweifach, B. W., Nagler, A. L. and Thomas, L. (1956). The role of epinephrine in the reactions produced by the endotoxins of gram-negative bacteria. *Journal of Experimental Medicine* **104**: 881–889.

5

Acute Intestinal Failure

Introduction

By 'acute intestinal failure' is meant necrosis, threatened or complete, of the part of the alimentary tract supplied by the superior mesenteric artery. This event is becoming increasingly frequent. Figure 5.1 illustrates the certification rate in England and Wales over the last decade, and most countries which record reliable medical statistics will produce similar figures. The extent of the problem is underestimated, however, because of accidents of terminology. If an operation or an autopsy demonstrates mechanical blockage of a major visceral artery, the death will be recorded as due to intestinal infarction, but if no such block is found, another diagnostic label will be given.

There is here a difficulty, because in only a small (and indeed diminishing) proportion of intestinal infarctions is there an embolus in the vessel. In about one-third of the reported cases the major arteries are quite normal and patent.[57, 83, 104, 105] In others, the vessels may be narrowed by atheroma, even sometimes to the point of total occlusion, but it is well recognized[25, 33, 36, 103] that such lesions are often quite asymptomatic so that the actual infarction must have been precipitated by some additional factor. It follows therefore that where an infarcted intestine is found in the presence of a healthy arterial tree which has suddenly become blocked by an embolus, the logical sequence:

ARTERIAL BLOCK – ISCHAEMIA – INFARCTION – DEATH

applies, but in other instances the fatal event is less easy to determine. The classical description of mesenteric embolism related to the young patient with mitral valve disease and atrial fibrillation who presented with the dramatic onset of abdominal pain which was followed by the development of peritoneal signs. This is a clinical situation which nowadays is practically never encountered. The presence or absence of an occlusion in the major vessels is impossible to determine by clinical means, and indeed is not always relevant to treatment. For this reason the terms 'mesenteric embolus', 'mesenteric thrombosis' and 'non-occlusive infarction' have to an extent lost their value, and 'acute intestinal failure' is preferred.

Nomenclature

The syndrome has been recognized for many years and has been described with a variety of names such as:

apoplexies viscérales[50]

postoperative enterocolitis[109]
enteritis necroticans[106, 109, 137]
agnogenic infarction[10]
darmbrand[51]
pseudomembranous enterocolitis[60, 75]
haemorrhagic enterocolitis[135]
acute necrotizing enterocolitis[62, 71, 117]
intestinal infarction without vascular lesion[48, 59, 77, 83, 101]
haemorrhagic duodenitis and ileitis[70]
entérites ischémiques aigües[114]
non-specific enteritis[42]
acute haemorrhagic necrosis[34, 98, 125, 126]
necrotizing enteropathy[34]
acute haemorrhage and necrosis of intestine[44]
non-occlusive infarction[10, 41, 52, 53, 88, 105, 116]
non-thrombotic intestinal infarction[52]
non-obstructive mesenteric arterial insufficiency[18]
pig-bel[100]
terminal haemorrhagic necrosing enteropathy (THNE)[12]

Each author who has devised a new terminology for his (usually small) series of cases has acted in the apparent belief that he was reporting a new disease. It is quite obvious, however, on studying the literature as a whole, that what is being described is the response of the intestine, as a target organ, to a variety of rather similar challenges. The subject was reviewed by the author in 1962.[91] Our understanding of the mechanisms underlying intestinal failure has been hampered by preoccupation with major vascular occlusion. With the realization of the unique behaviour of the mucosal circulation under circumstances of stress (see Chapters 3 and 4), much that has in the past seemed muddled and obscure, in fact falls into place.

Factors leading to acute intestinal failure

Factors leading to acute intestinal failure (Fig. 5.2) may be thought of as:

1. *Deficiencies in major blood flow*, as determined by the cardiac output or by local conditions in the major mesenteric arteries (see Chapter 2).
2. Factors operating *within the wall of the bowel*. These include radial muscular tension, and local tissue sensitivities leading to focal reactions such as the Arthus[47] and Schwartzmann phenomena. Among these may also be included pharmacological agents such as digitalis, and pressor amines which act on the bowel wall and its small vessels (see Chapter 3).
3. *Intraluminal factors*. These include:
   (a) tryptic activity and other influences which imperil the integrity of the mucosal barrier, and
   (b) the bacterial flora.

The bowel is unique in that it is normally populated by pathogenic bacteria which are capable of producing endotoxins and exotoxins possessing intense physiological potency. Any weakening of the mucosal defences will permit invasion to occur, resulting in local inflammation and generalized

DEATHS FROM ARTERIAL EMBOLISM AND THROMBOSIS OF MESENTERIC ARTERY
ENGLAND AND WALES   1967 - 1973

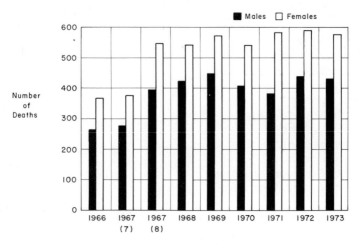

Note :   ICD No. 7 th Revision 570·2
8 th Revision 444·2

DEATHS FROM MESENTERIC INFARCTION
ENGLAND AND WALES   1973

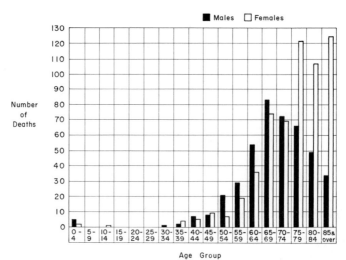

Figure 5.1. The incidence of death from intestinal infarction: (a) by year; (b) by age group. (Registrar General's figures for England and Wales, 1966–1973)

circulatory effects. Whether a sufficiently virulent strain of bacteria can invade a healthy gut with normal vasculature is a matter of dispute, but there is evidence that in certain circumstances this can occur (see below).

REDUCED BLOOD FLOW

FALL IN
CARDIAC
OUTPUT

EMBOLUS OR
THROMBUS

ALTERED
LUMINAL
CONTENTS

Bacteria (clostridia)
Mucin Barrier (tryptic
activity)

LIMITING FACTORS IN BOWEL WALL

Increased Radial Tension (obstruction)

Local Sensitivity reactions
(Arthus, Schwartzmann)

Vasoconstrictors (digitalis)

Specific causes of acute intestinal failure

Mesenteric embolus and thrombosis

Previously recognized as a frequent complication of atrial fibrillation, congenital cardiac defects or endocardial thrombosis, mesenteric embolus has now become a rare disease. It is none the less of very considerable scientific and academic interest, because it is the nearest approach in the human being to the situation which the experimental scientist produces by occluding the SMA of a healthy animal. A very complete study of the clinical

Table 5.1 Superior mesenteric embolectomy—published successes

Reference	Sex and age of patient	Interval between onset and operation	Concomitant bowel resection	Postoperative course
Shaw & Rutledge, 1957[123]	F/54	8 hours	—	'Second look' at 24 hours (no resection necessary). Postoperative aortogram at 80 days confirmed patency
Miller & di Mare, 1958[97]	M/49	8 hours	70 cm ileum	Uneventful
Stewart et al., 1960[127]	M/65	'Several hours'	21 cm ileum	Death at 5 years
	M/59	24 hours	18 cm jejunum	Diarrhoea and bleeding 1 week
Saris & Uricchio, 1960[118]	M/47	26 hours	Nil	Uneventful
Atwell, 1961[5]	M/18	24 hours	Nil	'Second look' at 24 hours (no resection necessary)
Senn et al., 1961[121]	M/32	24 hours	25 cm ileum	Uneventful
Zuidema et al., 1961[141]	F/57	3½ hours	Nil	'Second look' at 24 hours (no resection necessary)
de Niord & Ring, 1961[32]	F/34	24 hours	Nil	Jejunal stenosis and malabsorption
Chalnot et al., 1962[27]	F/61	28 hours	Nil	Uneventful
Martinis, 1962[95]	Not given	25 hours	Nil	Uneventful
Hardy, 1963[55]	F/63	4½ hours	Nil	Uneventful
Baue & Austen, 1963[6]	M/63	4 hours+	Nil	Uneventful

of arteriotomy

	M/26	4 hours +	Nil	Diarrhoea and bleeding. Death at 3 months
Todd & Pearson, 1963[130]	F/57	48 hours	⅓ of small bowel	Uneventful
Allgower, 1963[3]	M/47	17 hours	Nil	Uneventful
Bohn & Carroll, 1964[15]	M/64	3½ hours	Nil	Uneventful
Olsen & Santer, 1965[102]	F/72	4 hours	Nil	Death at 6 weeks (pulmonary embolus)
Kreager, 1965[81A]	M/47	29 hours	Nil	Uneventful
Bergan et al., 1969[1,8,9]	M/53	6 hours	Nil	Uneventful. Well at 2 years
	F/55	6 hours	Nil	Pulmonary oedema, malabsorption. Well at 5 years
	M/36	18 hours	Nil	—
Jago, 1971[61]	F/57	4 hours	Nil initially	Resection for jejunal obstruction at 2 months
Sasser, 1971[119]	M/66	20 hours	30 cm jejunum	Uneventful
	M/55	22 hours	50 cm jejunum	Death from pulmonary embolus
Wangensteen et al., 1972[131A]	M/61	2½ hours	Nil	Uneventful
Skinner et al., 1974[125]	F/47	6 hours	Nil	Uneventful
McKenzie & Provan, 1974[89]	F/50	6 hours	Nil	'Second look' at 24 hours. Death at 19 months
Schoofs et al., 1975[120]	M/73	24 hours	Nil	Wound infection. Well at 2 months

literature was reported in 1941 by Bowen and Felger,[17] which accurately defined the position at that time. Their analysis of 1,142 reported cases of occlusion of the mesenteric vessels revealed the following features:

1. The usual end-results of either an arterial or a venous occlusion was a haemorrhagic infarct of the bowel. The site of the vascular block was not always ascertainable either clinically or at post-mortem.

2. Arterial occlusion (51 per cent of the total) was slightly commoner than venous occlusion (43 per cent). Occlusion of both arteries and veins was unusual (6 per cent).

3. Venous occlusion was usually secondary to peritoneal sepsis, portal hypertension or blood dyscrasia.

4. The SMA was involved 40 times as frequently as the IMA. (It should be emphasized that this was a clinical finding. Later autopsy studies have shown that in fact the IMA is more frequently occluded than the SMA, but that this is usually asymptomatic because of the excellent collateral network to the colon.[24, 31, 65]

5. Embolism was more common than thrombosis as a cause of arterial occlusion.

6. Perforation and sloughing of the bowel were rare, death usually occurring before this took place.

7. The over-all mortality, at that time, given all available methods of treatment, was 86 per cent. It was almost 100 per cent in unoperated cases, although the occasional spontaneous resolution did occur. There were 116 recorded survivors following resection, of whom 90 had undergone removal of less than 200 cm of intestine, and 26 had had more than this removed.

The authors concluded that immediate operation with resection of non-viable gut was the treatment of choice in all cases of mesenteric vascular occlusion, and this view was generally held until Klass in 1951 published the first technically successful embolectomy.[71] His patient, a 64-year-old man, who suffered from rheumatic heart disease and auricular fibrillation, developed sudden abdominal pain, vomiting and shock, and 14 hours after the onset of his illness an embolus was removed from the origin of the SMA. Death occurred 48 hours later from acute left ventricular failure, but at autopsy the bowel was found to be viable.

The first SMA embolectomy to be followed by survival was performed by Stewart the same year, and reported by Stewart *et al.* in 1960.[127] There have since been many successful operations reported, performed at intervals of from 12 to 96 hours following the infarction (Table 5.1). Glotzer and Shaw,[45] in an autopsy study designed to assess the potential of reconstructive surgery, found that, of 20 patients dying from acute SMA occlusion, 13 would have been amenable to direct attack on the blocked vessel, 4 would probably have survived following bowel resection, and only 3 showed evidence of spreading thrombosis, which would have made operation impossible. Of 3 long-standing occlusions, 2 were potentially reconstructable and 1 resectable. Ottinger and Austen[104] came to a similar conclusion. It is important to note that, even in patients who succumb, viability is usually restored to the bowel, and death occurs from causes other than sloughing and peritonitis.

The relative frequency of embolus and thrombosis is not easy to determine, but there appears not unexpectedly to have been a steady decline in the incidence of emboli over the last two decades.

Johnson and Baggenstoss[66] outlined stringent criteria for the diagnosis of mesenteric embolism, namely:

1. There must be a source for an embolus.
2. There must be clinical symptoms of sudden onset.
3. A short section only of the SMA must be involved.
4. The microscopic appearance of the occlusion must suggest an embolus.
5. Embolic phenomena must have occurred elsewhere.

Applying these criteria, they found that an embolus accounted for 19 out of 45 cases seen at the Mayo Clinic between 1911 and 1949. If, however, the diagnosis of mesenteric embolus depended on such findings, which can only be verified post mortem, the reported incidence would be deceptively low. None the less, although some authors have recently shown an equal or even preponderant number of emboli as against thromboses,[2, 5, 13, 26, 49, 89, 140] the general tendency has suggested that other forms of acute intestinal failure do, in fact, predominate.[14, 20, 41, 52, 68, 78, 104, 125] We now recognize that the relative frequency of embolus and thrombosis is an artificial statistic in that a mesenteric arterial block bears little time relation to clinical events. The unique importance of the mesenteric embolus is that it is a condition which, if diagnosed early, is curable—which cannot be said of any other type of acute mesenteric vascular disease.

Atheromatous ulceration, with consequent platelet accretion, is very commonly found at the origin of the superior mesenteric artery. Clearly, this on occasion will lead to acute occlusion of the lumen, with subsequent death of the bowel, in the same way that acute occlusion of a stenotic femoral artery can precipitate gangrene in the foot. The analogy, however, is not so simple. Not only can stenosis or occlusion of the SMA be present without causing any symptoms, but also, as has been already pointed out, the bowel can become infarcted in spite of there being a perfectly normal and patent vascular tree. It is therefore quite wrong to conclude that a patient with an infarcted bowel and a blocked SMA has sustained a recent acute thrombosis—the block may have been there for months or even years, and the intestinal failure has occurred through a fall in cardiac output, a local Schwartzmann phenomenon or other unrelated cause. This is not to say that the occlusion should be ignored and no attempt made to restore patency—this is far from being the case, for the reasons given above. However, all reported evidence goes to show that the results of surgery for 'acute thrombosis' are much worse than when an embolus is present.

Low-flow states

Cases of intestinal failure which are not due to mechanical blockage of the major arteries have, as already explained, been classified under a variety of different names, the most all-embracing of which is the term 'non-occlusive infarction' (see above). The great majority of these patients have in common some central factor which results in diminished cardiac output and mesenteric flow. The more important of these factors which have been described are as follows.

Congestive cardiac failure is a common and important predisposing cause of intestinal failure.[37, 61] Kligerman's[78] series reports that 75 of 109 patients in intestinal failure were also in heart failure. Renton[116] reviewed the literature up to that time and showed that 220 patients out of the 284 (77 per cent) reported had severe heart disease, including acute or chronic congestive failure and a history of myocardial infarction and angina. About half the patients were in atrial fibrillation or other arrhythmia; the importance of arrhythmia in reducing cardiac output and precipitating intestinal damage has been underlined by Britt and Cheek,[19] who were able in the experimental laboratory to demonstrate an abrupt fall in mesenteric flow following induced atrial fibrillation. Other authors[63] have demonstrated a drop in mesenteric blood flow during paroxysmal atrial tachycardia, and have described areas of ischaemia and necrosis of the bowel in such cases.

The role which digitalis has to play in this situation is uncertain. It is well documented[107] that digitalis and similar glycosides have a selective vasoconstrictive action on the mesenteric circulation, and many of the clinical series reported contain a high proportion of patients suffering from digitalis overdosage.[41, 111, 130] However, the local effect of digitalis on the bowel is often counterbalanced by the control which the drug exercises on left ventricular failure, with a corresponding rise in cardiac output. Certainly, intestinal failure is not confined to patients who are on digitalis, and has been reported in those who have stopped taking it.[41] Another factor which frequently operates in these patients is the haemoconcentration which follows administration of rapidly acting diuretic agents.[122]

Trauma and 'shock'

As described in Chapter 2, the intestinal lesion shock is very much a fact in the dog, and haemorrhagic necrosis of the alimentary tract is frequent following the challenge of oligaemia, trauma or endotoxaemia. It has been known since the classical work of Wiggers[134] and of Fine[40] that experimentally induced shock in the exsanguinated dog becomes irreversible due to the development of intestinal necrosis. If the shed blood is returned to the animal before the bowel lesion has had time to develop (that is to say, within about 90 minutes) recovery ensues, but if transfusion is delayed for 4 hours the cardiac output inexorably falls away, and no treatment is effective. The unique role of the mesenteric circulation in the development of irreversible shock was further demonstrated by Lillehei,[85, 86] who showed that selective perfusion of the SMA prevented irreversibility in a way that perfusion of other crucial arterial pathways did not.

There are, however, considerable species differences in the intestinal response to shock, and the rabbit, cat and monkey behave quite differently from the dog which, perhaps unfortunately, is the experimental animal most accessible to human researchers. The clinical counterpart to the experimental canine lesion, if it exists, does not appear to be of fundamental importance. Clinical experience accumulated from two World Wars and from the Korean and Vietnam conflicts have produced no convincing evidence that intestinal necrosis is an important cause of death in fit human beings who have lost blood because of wounding.

There is none the less a small body of clinical evidence which suggests that intestinal failure can on occasion follow trauma. Thus Renton[116] described the case of a fit 18-year-old male who developed necrosis of the entire bowel from the upper jejunum to the pelvic colon 24 hours following a traffic accident involving multiple fractures. There was no intra-abdominal injury and no occlusion of any intestinal vessel. More recently, Haglund and his associates[54] in Göteborg have described haemorrhagic mucosal lesions with epithelial lifting, entirely characteristic of mucosal ischaemia, in a series of 7 patients suffering from varying degrees of circulatory depletion. Three of their patients in fact had occlusive infarction of the gut in areas distant to the mucosal lesion, and should probably be excluded on these grounds. The other 4 patients however, had no such problem, and may be considered to be pure examples of the intestinal shock lesion. This is the first time that this lesion has been described in man.

Haemoconcentration and intravascular coagulation

Fogarty and Fletcher[41] have emphasized the importance of the haematocrit in the genesis of intestinal failure. They pointed out that haematocrit is substantially higher in patients who develop necrosis in the absence of arterial occlusion, and emphasize that a lowered cardiac output coupled with rising blood viscosity will inevitably lead to a fall in mesenteric flow. This point has been further emphasized by Sharefkin and Silen[122] with regard to diuretic agents.

Whitehead[132, 133] has shown that intestinal failure is frequently associated with the presence of microthrombi in other organs such as lungs and kidneys, and has many of the features now known to be characteristic of disseminated intravascular coagulation. The factors which precipitate this syndrome in man are far from being completely understood, but include multiple trauma (as may have been the case in Renton's patient), severe burns, septicaemia and anaphylaxis. The Schwartzmann reaction, which is a manifestation of sensitivity to gram-negative endotoxin, is another potent cause of disseminated intravascular coagulation (DIC), and a generalized Schwartzmann reaction could well be an important factor in the causation of intestinal failure. Indeed, a similar lesion can be produced in rabbits, by injecting a small sensitizing dose of endotoxin into the colonic wall, and following this up with a larger dose intravenously.[11] Bearing in mind the constant high level of endotoxin in the intestinal lumen, it is easy to see how this situation could occur clinically.

Perhaps arising from a similar mechanism, intestinal necrosis has been reported[108, 110, 113] as occurring as a complication of renal transplantation. It usually affects patients who have had a difficult post-transplantation course, with high doses of immunosuppressive agents and repeated episodes of rejection. Whether the intestinal lesion is a result of tissue sensitization following the transplant, or whether the immunosuppressive therapy lowers mucosal resistance to bacterial invasion, remains undecided.

Abnormalities of the bowel wall

Dilatation of the lumen of the bowel due to a distal obstruction will cause a corresponding fall-off in mucosal flow (see Chapter 3) and, if sufficiently severe and prolonged, may precipitate necrosis. An example of this is the ischaemic colitis which occurs above an obstructing carcinoma. However, the damage is usually focal and the cause obvious (see Chapter 8). Similar acute and massive necrosis has been described in association with rheumatoid arthritis, polyarteritis and diabetes. Although it is difficult to be absolutely sure that these are not in fact examples of mechanical infarction due to small vessel involvement, it does seem that on occasion massive necrosis, out of all proportion to the local vascular lesion and in apparently normal parts of the bowel, may occur.[90, 104]

Anthony[1] has described sudden unexpected intestinal necrosis as a complication of functioning carcinoid tumour, and speculates that this is due to bradykinin and 5-hydroxytryptamine, secreted by the tumour and conveyed in the intestinal lymphatics.

The contents of the bowel

Under normal circumstances (given, that is, a normal blood supply) the intestinal mucosa is well able to resist bacterial challenge, and when organisms such as Clostridia are found within the wall of the gut, they are there as secondary invaders. None the less, these organisms produce powerfully constrictive exotoxins, and the question arises as to whether the balance between bacterial aggression and mucosal defence can ever be shifted the other way; that is to say, whether an organism of unusual virulence can invade a mucosa which has a normal vascularity. There is evidence that this can in fact occur. In 1949 two groups in north Germany[39, 138] reported a series of patients who had developed sudden and unexplained necrosis of the small bowel, usually the jejunum. A strain of *C. welchii* (type F) isolated from these patients was, beyond reasonable doubt, the causative organism. A similar condition had previously been reported under the name 'darmbrand',[51] in which the same clostridium had been found. In 1959 Fethers[38] reported a further 3 cases of clostridial infection of the bowel, all of them fatal, as a complication of gastrointestinal haemorrhage. Killingback and Lloyd Williams[73] described a condition of 'necrotizing enterocolitis', and in their 6 patients there was no alteration of the mesenteric vascular supply but all showed large numbers of gram-positive rods in the mucosa and deeper layers of the bowel. Murrell and Roth,[99, 100] working in the highlands of New Guinea, described a necrotizing enteritis of the jejunum occurring following the ingestion of partially-cooked pork, and associated with the presence in the bowel of another type of clostridium (type C). This condition, known as 'pig-bel' varies from a fulminating massive gangrene to a relatively trivial form of gastroenteritis. Interestingly, an intermediate type was described (type 3) resulting in acute and chronic obstruction caused by scarring stenosis and fistula formation. This spectrum of change is quite typical of focal ischaemia in the small and large intestine (see Chapters 3 and 9). A further 6 cases of clostridial gangrene were reported from Sydney by Renwick *et al.*[117]

Leaving aside the cases reported from Britain, in whom there might well have been underlying atheromatous lesions of the main arteries, or cardiac decompensation, with secondary invasion by clostridia, patients suffering from necrotizing enterocolitis are of all ages, and include many young people and children, who would not be expected to have any intrinsic vascular disease. This applies particularly to the cases reported from Australia and New Guinea, and on this evidence one must conclude that the normal gastrointestinal tract can undergo ischaemic necrosis provided that the invading organism is of sufficient virulence. The type C (or F) clostridium produces an enterotoxin which seems capable of inducing intense mucosal vasoconstriction, and may cause necrosis in the absence of any pre-existing vascular lesion.

Tryptic activity

As well as the bacterial content, the chemical contents of the bowel exert a strong influence on its behaviour, following any type of ischaemic challenge. The first, and perhaps the most important, line of defence is the mucous barrier which coats the epithelium, and there is some experimental evidence (see Chapter 4) that haemorrhagic necrosis of the gut as seen in the experimentally shocked animal occurs from tryptic digestion of this mucus, so that proteolytic enzymes can penetrate to the mucosa, in which the lysosomes have been damaged by ischaemia, and lay it open to bacterial invasion. Prior use of an elemental diet which reduces or abolishes this tryptic activity has been shown[16] to confer some protection against standard ischaemic injury. While at present there is no information on the clinical relevance of these findings, it would seem likely that the mucosal barrier provides the same protection in man as it does in the experimental animal.

The aortoiliac steal syndrome

By a 'steal' is meant redistribution of flow from one vascular bed into another, due to a pressure gradient created by a stenosis between the two respective arteries of supply. The first such syndrome to be described was the 'subclavian steal' in which a block in the subclavian artery creates a head of pressure between the circulations to the brain and the arm, so that blood flows out of the circle of Willis, retrogradely down the vertebral artery and so into the subclavian beyond the block.[115] The existence of a similar state of affairs in the mesenteric circulation has been postulated,[30, 135] and the term 'aortoiliac steal' has been used to describe two different sets of circumstances.

1. Ischaemia of the legs may occur in the postabsorption period. As described in Chapter 3, ingestion of food leads to an increase in blood flow to the SMA, which normally is attained by a rise in cardiac output. If, however, the cardiac reserve is diminished, or there is an occlusion of the aorta, then the compensatory mechanisms may fail. Harris and Charlesworth[56] describe a patient with a complete aortic occlusion involving the inferior mesenteric artery, whose legs were supplied by a meandering mesenteric artery. She experienced severe pain in the buttock on eating, unless she ate her food lying in bed. A Dacron bypass completely relieved her symptoms. Brooks and Bron[21] describe a patient with a similar lesion whose claudication distance was reduced from 100 to 5 metres following a meal, at which time he also experienced pain and numbness of the left foot. Again, successful arterial reconstruction abolished the symptoms. This situation appears very uncommon, and the cases are of anecdotal interest.

2. Of much greater importance is the situation whereby the iliofemoral circulation appears to 'steal' blood from the bowel.

Kountz *et al.*[80] reported a series of patients who died from intestinal infarction following sympathectomy and/or reconstructive aortoiliac surgery. This was particularly likely to occur in patients with occlusive disease of the mesenteric arteries, and the authors' view was that it was the result of reflex vasoconstriction in the gut vessels rather than simple mechanical redistribution of blood following the surgery. Experiments on dogs demonstrated that lumbar sympathectomy increased flow and lowered resistance in the legs, but had the opposite effect on the gut. Subsequent authors[28, 81, 136] have suggested that it is the opening up of the vessels in the legs which causes a direct steal of blood.

It is clearly very important to know whether restoration of blood supply to the legs by sympathectomy or arterial surgery is likely to infarct the bowel. It may be said that, for a number of reasons, this seems not to be the case. In the first place, small bowel ischaemia following aortic surgery is excessively rare, amounting to less than 1 per cent[67] (this does not, of course, take into account colonic damage resulting from sacrifice of the inferior mesenteric artery, which is discussed below and is a quite separate problem). Secondly, it is well recognized that acute intestinal failure can follow any sort of surgery, even haemorrhoidectomy,[28] or no surgery at all, and many patients undergoing arterial operations will have the sort of cardiac history which is the normal background to this event. Finally, study of the haemodynamics of steal syndromes in general, and of subclavian steal in particular, has cast considerable doubt on their validity except as angiographic curiosities.[28] Theoretical analysis of the likely consequences of increasing flow in the distal aorta[129] suggests that, given a normal cardiac output, even very large increases would not affect SMA perfusion pressure (and hence mesenteric flow) unless there were gross aortic obstruction above the origins of the mesenteric vessels, as in a coarctation. It has been calculated[129] that quadrupling the flow to the legs would 'steal' about 8 ml/min from the mesenteric circulation,[128] and most arterial operations do little more than double the flow, and then only transiently. Where, however, cardiac reserve is diminished so that output cannot rise if the peripheral resistance is lowered, and particularly if there is a coexistent stenosis of the SMA, then this may not apply, and shutdown may occur.

On the whole, the consensus of evidence suggests that the iliofemoral circulation does not divert blood from the bowel, either during exercise or following operation, unless there is a combination of diminished cardiac output and local abnormality in the mesenteric circulation. It is questionable whether this is fairly described as a 'steal' syndrome.

The clinical picture

Intestinal failure is primarily a condition of older people, as would be expected from its association with degenerative cardiovascular disease. Renton's[116] review of 227 patients suffering from 'non-occlusive infarction', found the mean age to be 71, with males and females equally affected.

Acute failure is frequently preceded by a prodromal period of chronic or episodic abdominal pain, usually related to meals and sometimes associated with diarrhoea and loss of weight.[9, 10, 72, 94] Whether this pain is true 'intestinal angina' (see Chapter 6), or whether it is due to repeated small infarcts or to transient episodes of low intestinal blood flow secondary to alterations in cardiac output, cannot at present be determined.

History

The *onset* of the condition is usually abrupt, but may be insidious. Very often the patient is already under treatment in hospital for associated cardiac, respiratory or renal problems, so that the initial complaint of vague abdominal pain may not be seen as representing a new development in the illness, and so escape documentation. None the less, abdominal pain is invariably present, and is generally colicky in nature at the outset and ill localized. As the condition progresses, the pain becomes constant unremitting, and is felt first in the right iliac fossa and then over the entire abdomen. *Diarrhoea* is usual, and frequently the motions contain altered blood (it would seem likely that occult blood, if looked for, would be almost universally present). *Vomiting* occurs in about one-third of cases, but haematemesis is rare.

Examination of the abdomen

In the early stages of the illness, examination of the abdomen is quite negative. In fact, as has been pointed out by many authors, the distress of the patient is out of all proportion to the physical signs which can be elicited. Apart from slight tenderness in the right iliac fossa and some exaggeration of the bowel sounds, there may be nothing to find. As the illness develops over the course of hours or (more usually) one to two days, the abdomen becomes distended and silent, with gross tenderness and a positive rebound sign, at the same time as the signs of peripheral circulatory failure begin to appear. There is pallor, anxiety, sweating, tachypnoea and air-hunger, later followed by cyanosis, hypotension and anuria. The clinical picture suggests a fulminating abdominal catastrophe such as a leaking aneurysm, hyperacute pancreatitis or perforation of a hollow viscus. By the time obvious signs of surgical illness have begun to appear, the patient is almost certainly beyond the point of recovery, so that it is essential to make the diagnosis at an early stage. However, in the absence of any specific test for acute intestinal ischaemia, clinical impression remains the most useful means of establishing it.

Endoscopy: there are a few clinical[23] and laboratory[93] accounts of the appearances seen on conventional rigid sigmoidoscopic examination. The mucosa is engorged, and raised into irregular bluish projections, with oedema, contact bleeding and ulceration. There may be blood and mucus coming down from above the instrument. So far, there is no reported information on the use of the fibreoptic colonoscope in this situation.

A peritoneal tap almost always produces blood-stained fluid, and is a useful diagnostic test.[69]

Laboratory data

It must be admitted that the clinical laboratory has little help to offer towards making the diagnosis. All are agreed that the leucocyte count is raised early in the course of the disease, so that a finding of 20,000 or 30,000 leucocytes in the peripheral blood, especially if the abdominal signs are unimpressive, should prompt the suspicion of intestinal ischaemia.

Serum enzyme concentrations have proved a surprisingly disappointing index as to the existence or severity of bowel necrosis.[139] The best data we have on this problem are those accumulated by Vyden,[13] who carried out a detailed biochemical study in Australia of 12 patients with acute mesenteric vascular insufficiency.

Radiological appearances

The appearances on the plain x-ray progress from the complete absence of gas patterns as seen on early films to dilated loops with multiple fluid levels in the advanced stage of the disease. Various radiologists have described intramural thickening, and abnormal separation of the gas-filled intestinal loops in the early stages of intestinal ischaemia,[13] but these appearances have not been verified in a practical context. One radiological sign should be mentioned for the purposes of completeness, which is the presence of gas bubbles in the portal vein, which is diagnostic of intestinal necrosis;[128] but this radiological sign is of mainly academic interest as, at the time of writing, no adult patient who has exhibited it has survived the experience.

The place of emergency aortography.

Aakhus,[1] Williams[135] and Kieny[72] have emphasized the great importance of an immediate aortogram to differentiate between occlusive and non-occlusive bowel infarction. Indeed, an aortogram will immediately make this distinction, but in practice, because intestinal failure is so difficult to diagnose clinically, this is seldom the question that is being asked! The opponents of aortography argue as follows.

1. It is now widely recognized (see above) that varying degrees of occlusion of the visceral arteries are quite commonly encountered in normal human beings over the age of 45, and often are without any demonstrable effect upon their health. It therefore follows that the angiographic demonstration of a blocked mesenteric artery in a patient with indeterminate abdominal pain gives little guidance as to when the occlusion occurred or whether it is the cause of the symptoms.

2. Failure to show such a block is of no diagnostic help to the surgeon and, if signs of peritonitis are present, will not and should not deter him from exploring the abdomen. Some authors have claimed[19] that intestinal failure, threatened or complete, can be diagnosed on the aortogram by the presence of a narrowed distal arterial tree with spasm of the intramural vessels. The situation can then be treated by epidural blockade or instilla-

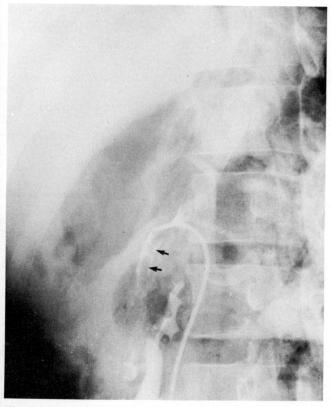

Fig. 5.3. Selective SMA angiogram, showing a mesenteric embolus (by courtesy of Dr Hans Herlinger).

tion of vasodilator substances such as glucagon into the superior mesenteric artery, and an unnecessary laparotomy avoided. While this is a most attractive proposition, which may well point the way to future developments in this field, there is at present very scanty clinical evidence on which to base such a treatment policy. Most experienced surgeons agree that the aortographic appearances are far from specific, and that if doubt exists it is safer to operate.

When a new diagnostic facility is provided, it tends at first to be used without particular regard to its effectiveness. If aortography (which is, after all, an expensive procedure, and not without risk) is made available for emergency diagnosis of abdominal pain, a degree of abuse is inevitable.

Having said all this it must in fairness be admitted that when embarking on an operation for suspected mesenteric vascular occlusion, most surgeons would be pleased to have an aortogram available!

The pathology of acute intestinal failure

Ischaemia of the midgut, induced by ligation of the superior mesenteric artery, has been extensively studied in the laboratory, and an account of the main findings was given in Chapter 4. Chiu *et al.*[27A] have graded the changes observed in the mucosa as follows:

Grade 0:   normal villi
Grade 1:   development of a subepithelial space (Grunhagen's space) at the apex of the villus
Grade 2:   the extension of the space, with lifting of the epithelial layer from the lamina propria
Grade 3:   massive epithelial lifting down the sides of the villus, with denudation of some of the tips
Grade 4:   complete denudation of the villi, with lamina propria and dilated capillaries exposed
Grade 5:   digestion and disintegration of the lamina propria, with haemorrhage and ulceration

A detailed study using the electron microscope suggested that the fluid in the subepithelial space originated partly from the capillary but also from the lumen of the bowel.

The authors were able to correlate the speed of development of mucosal damage with blood flow in the SMA (Fig. 5.4). With complete occlusion of the SMA, grade 5 mucosal damage was achieved in some instances within 30 minutes.

As ischaemia progresses, more obvious and gross lesions become apparent. The superficial capillaries dilate and bleed into the wall and lumen of the bowel, which becomes progressively more oedematous. An inflammatory response of polymorphs accumulates and eventually necrosis spreads from the mucosa out to the serosa so that the whole bowel becomes frankly gangrenous, its colour varying from a dark green to black. Changes are usually most marked in the ileocaecal area, which is the part of the

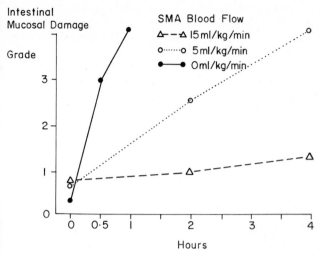

Fig. 5.4. The relationship between SMA flow and pace of mucosal damage. (Reproduced from C. J. Chiu, (1976), *Archives of Surgery*, **101**: 480 by kind permission of the author and the editor.)

bowel embryologically and anatomically most distant from the blood supply.

In many instances the bowel appears normal from the outside, though it may be slightly reddened or darkened, whereas the mucosa is haemorrhagic and the intestinal contents purulent. Mucosal changes vary from discrete ragged ulcers to complete denudation. Adherent or sloughed membranous material is often seen, intact or divided into small islands: the so-called 'pseudomembranous enterocolitis' (Fig. 5.5). In the same patient a mixture of haemorrhage, ulceration and pseudomembrane formation may be seen, the distribution of the lesions bearing no particular relationship to the main arteries and veins. Microscopically, the capillaries and small veins contain thrombi, and similar thrombi[132, 133] are found in other organs, particularly the lungs and kidneys, which is characteristic of disseminated intravascular coagulation (DIC). The relationship is complex, because there is evidence both that acute intestinal necrosis can lead to DIC and that DIC, perhaps secondary to a generalized Schwartzmann reaction (see above), can infarct the bowel.

Management

Any discussion of management of this condition is, in the nature of things, bound to be academic and theoretical because in practice the diagnosis is almost never made except on the operating table, when the true state of the patient comes as somewhat of a surprise. As already emphasized, the young patient with the 'classical' history of a mesenteric embolus is now a rarity. The usual clinical picture is entirely non-specific, and consists simply in acute abdominal pain with peripheral circulatory collapse. However, much the same type of preliminary resuscitation will have been used whether the operative diagnosis turns out to be pancreatitis, ischaemia or perforation, so that this diagnostic imprecision may in practical terms matter less than would seem.

Having made this point, it may be useful to consider the management

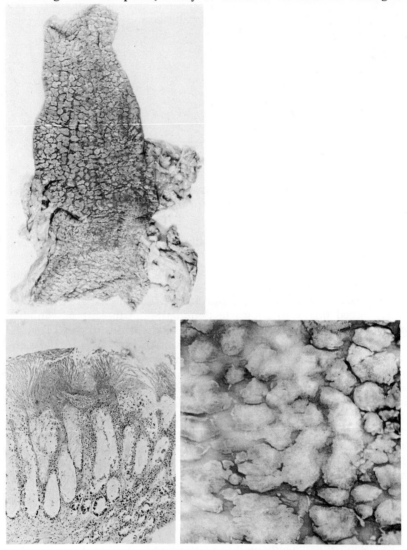

Fig. 5.5 Pseudomembranous enterocolitis (by courtesy of Dr V. J. McGovern).

of a theoretical case in which the diagnosis of intestinal failure had been made preoperatively.

Figure 4.8 demonstrates the physiological consequences of massive acute ischaemia of the bowel. It will be seen that they stem from, on the one hand, loss of fluid into the wall and lumen of the gut and, on the other, from the effects of bacterial invasion. Therapy should therefore logically be directed against both these life-threatening processes.

Fluid loss

Fluid loss is initially of water, electrolyte and protein. This results in a rise in haematocrit and blood viscosity with a fall in circulating volume, leading to impaired tissue flow in the gut wall itself and in the rest of the body. Experimentally, enormous losses of fluid can be recorded following ligation of the SMA,[92] but in the clinical situation these losses will have been mitigated by treatment. It is not possible to calculate in man the actual size and nature of the deficit, but replacement can be provided by serial measurements of the haematocrit and central venous pressure. Depending on the patient's known cardiac status and reserve, liberal quantities of balanced salt solutions (Hartman or Ringer-lactate) and plasma or medium molecular weight dextran, are given, until the haematocrit falls to below 45 and the central venous pressure rises to +5–10 cm of saline. (The use of low molecular weight dextran has been advocated on theoretical grounds (see Chapter 4) because of its reputed enhancement of small vessel flow. However, it is likely that this agent acts more as a plasma volume expander, and in any case its usefulness is limited by (1) its short stay in the circulation, (2) its anticoagulant properties, and (3) its capacity for interfering with cross-matching of blood to be transfused.)

Bacterial invasion and toxaemia

These clearly demand the use of *antibiotics*. While it is known from laboratory studies (Chapter 4) that pretreament with oral or (better) parenteral antibiotic agents mitigates the effects of intestinal ischaemia, in the clinical context it is impossible to ensure that the antibiotic in fact reaches the site of the damage. Blood is taken for culture (it is almost always sterile) and the chosen drug then given intravenously. This will be either an aminoglycoside such as gentamicin, tobramycin or amikasin, or a cephalosporin such as cephaloridine or cephradine. The dose given will depend on the weight of the patient, the urine output and the serum concentration of the drug.

The patient is *heparinized* in order to prevent extension of thrombus in the mesenteric vessels and gut wall and, perhaps more important, to counteract disseminated intravascular coagulation. Full heparinization is achieved by the immediate intravenous injection of 20,000 i.u., supplemented by 10,000 to 15,000 i.u. six-hourly, or by continuous intravenous infusion. The only theoretical objection to heparin therapy is accentuation of the bleeding from the haemorrhagic infarct, but in fact the cause of the haemorrhage is more usually a consumptive coagulopathy, and anticoagulation diminishes rather than intensifies it. Theoretically, administration of a fibrinolytic inhibitor such as ε-amino caproic acid (EACA) or aprotinin, in combination with heparin, should prevent haemorrhage by inhibiting secondary fibrinolysis, but there is no clinical information on this type of therapy. In any event, should surgery become necessary, it is a simple matter to reverse the heparin with the appropriate dose of protamine.

Metabolic acidosis

This is brought about by the combination of low tissue perfusion, haemoconcentration, and absorption (via the peritoneal cavity and intestinal lymphatics) of the products of bacterial and gut necrosis. To this is added a respiratory component derived from impaired ventilation due to interference with respiratory movements and increased blood viscosity with intrapulmonary sludging. Measurements of base excess, pCO_2 and pH will guide the amount of bicarbonate therapy required. Given reasonably normal pulmonary and renal function, however, restoration of the circulating blood volume will do much to restore correct acid–base equilibrium.

Specific pharmacological agents

Laboratory evidence suggests that the use of α blocking agents such as phenoxybenzamine[7, 29, 88] or β stimulators such as isoprenaline (Chapter 4) increase flow in the mesenteric circuit and help to preserve viability. Again, there is little or no controlled clinical information, and it is somewhat doubtful if, in the presence of a mesenteric vascular occlusion or massive shut-down of the minute vessels, the drug is capable of penetrating to the gut wall. Additionally, the fall in blood pressure which these agents (particularly phenoxybenzamine) bring about may be long-standing and difficult to control. By contrast, the use of vasoconstrictor agents such as metaraminol or noradrenaline is obviously to be condemned. There is as yet no reported experience of the use of glucagon or dopamine (see Chapter 3) in this situation. Because of their reputed effect on lysosomal membrane stability, oxygen consumption, arterial resistance and complement fixation by endotoxin, the use of *corticosteroids*, in massive suprapharmacological doses, has been advocated.[86]

While attractive on theoretical grounds, there is once again no firm clinical information reported which would support a case one way or the other. In actual practice, most clinicians would admit that it is nowadays unusual for anyone to die from any form of 'shock' without the benefit of a gram or two of methylprednisolone!

Digitalis has already been mentioned and incriminated as a constrictor in the mesenteric circuit and hence is a possible cause of intestinal failure. Its cautious use may, none the less, be justified in the control of fast atrial fibrillation and congestive failure, as in these circumstances its effect will be to raise the cardiac output and enhance mesenteric blood flow.

Aortography

The arguments for and against emergency aortography have been discussed earlier in this chapter. If facilities are available, and there is a strong presumption of a mesenteric embolus being the cause of the trouble, and the condition of the patient allows, then a (retrograde transfemoral) aortogram with free and selective mesenteric injections should probably be done. General applicability of the procedure is quite another question.

One theoretical advantage of aortography may be that it can be put to therapeutic use. Thus McGregor *et al.*[88] were able to dilate the distal intestinal vessels of a 63-year-old male in acute intestinal failure, by intra-arterial tolazoline. They frankly admit that the condition of their patient deteriorated following this procedure and in fact he eventually died, but the therapeutic possibilities are none the less interesting.

The place of splanchnic block

Orr *et al.*[103] treated 2 patients, 1 with total and 1 with partial small bowel ischaemia, by infiltration of the coeliac and mesenteric plexuses with lignocaine, which in each case was followed by recovery. Some experimental confirmation of this was provided by Liavåg[84] in dogs. More recently, there have been one or two threads of clinical evidence that this procedure may be useful in human beings.

Operative management

With very few exceptions[58, 79] there is practically no example in the recorded literature of a patient surviving acute intestinal failure without operative relief. This is not to say that surgery is curative; indeed this is far from being the case. But the continued presence of any significant length of ischaemic intestine within the abdominal cavity is not compatible with life.

The abdomen is opened via a right paramedian incision, which gives good general access to the peritoneal contents, and through which, given upward and downward extension if necessary, any necessary manoeuvre can be carried out.

Immediately the peritoneal cavity is opened, the diagnosis becomes obvious. There is a small collection of plum-coloured peritoneal fluid, and the loops of intestine are expanded, with dilated capillaries and venules on their serosal surface. But the most telling diagnostic feature is the absolutely unmistakable smell of ischaemic intestine, impossible to describe, but once experienced, quite unforgettable. There is no need for a formal exploration of the abdominal contents as is carried out in a routine laparotomy; indeed, this might be positively harmful. A quick manual exploration of the supra- and infracolic compartments of the abdomen is done, to exclude some coexistent inoperable situation such as widespread cancer. Attention is then directed to the mesenteric vessels. A loop of ileum is withdrawn and the mesentery carefully inspected in order to check the presence of pulsatile flow. If necessary, a leaf of peritoneum is picked up and delicately incised, in order to expose the bare vessel. It is useful to adjust the operating light so as to obtain a pinpoint reflection, which gives a very sensitive index of pulsatility.

From this point on, there are two alternative courses.

1. *In spite of unequivocal intestinal ischaemia, the mesenteric vessels are pulsatile up to the margins of the bowel.* In these circumstances it is obvious that no major arterial blockage is present and that no vascular reconstruction will be needed. The entire small bowel from the duodenojejunal flexure to the ileo-caecal junction is gently and carefully threaded through the fingers, in order to identify any necrotic areas. Great conservatism is exercised over the question of resection. Only if a loop appears hopelessly infarcted or on the point of perforation is it resected, but when resection

is carried out it must be wide and generous, and free bleeding must be obtained from the upper and lower ends. Where the small bowel is concerned, primary anastomosis is safe. However, if any area of the colon requires removal, the ends must be exteriorized (see Chapter 8).

Having completed the inspection (and, if necessary, resection) of the small bowel, the origin of the coeliac axis, the root of the mesentery and the preaortic region around the origin of the inferior mesenteric artery are infiltrated with a long-acting anaesthetic agent such as Marcain. The abdomen is then closed in one layer of through-and-through Nylon sutures, and arrangements made to return the patient to the operating theatre the following day.

2. *The small vessels to the intestine are collapsed.* The situation is first of all verified by dividing a leaf of the mesenteric peritoneum and inspecting the vessel wall directly, and with reflected light. If it is confirmed that the small vessels are indeed non-pulsatile, it follows that there must be a mechanical occlusion in the SMA. Accordingly, the origin of this artery is carefully palpated and its wall assessed, in order to determine whether one is dealing with an embolus or a thrombosis. (This factor may well have been decided preoperatively on the basis of the history and physi-

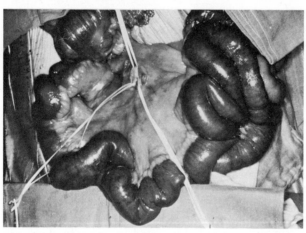

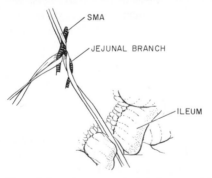

Fig. 5.6. Steps in mesenteric embolectomy: (1) Isolation of the SMA. (Photograph by courtesy of Mr R. W. Marcuson.)

cal signs). In either event, it is now clear that a vascular reconstruction must be attempted, unless the bowel is frankly gangrenous or perforated, which is exceedingly unusual.

Embolectomy is always worthwhile, and there are now a good number of successful reports in the literature. These are documented in Table 5.1. Where there is chronic obliterative disease, the situation is very different. As has already been emphasized, this is not simply a question of an acute thrombosis superimposed on a partially occluded vessel. The precipitating event which has caused failure of the intestine may well have been centrally rather than peripherally determined, and a technically successful reconstruction of the origin of the SMA may in fact be irrelevant to the physiological problem. It should none the less be attempted, because, as already stated, if nothing is done the patient will inevitably die.[76, 96]

Emergency revascularization of the gut

Direct attack on the origin of the SMA involves a dissection which is often difficult and prolonged, especially in an obese patient. Access is hampered by the portal vein, the neck of the pancreas with its many vascular connections, and the thick lymphatic tissues in the root of the mesentery. However, success can occasionally be achieved by this means, and in a thin patient it may be worth attempting a direct attack (Figs. 5.6–5.10).

An alternative method, and one which should normally be chosen by

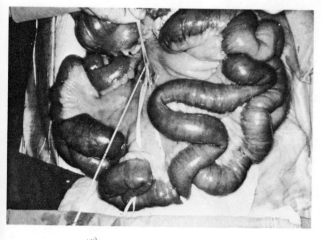

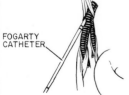

FOGARTY CATHETER

Fig. 5.7. Steps in mesenteric embolectomy: (2) introduction of the Fogarty catheter. (Photograph by courtesy of Mr R. W. Marcuson.)

the inexperienced surgeon, is illustrated in Fig. 5.11. It consists in expos-
ing the ileocolic artery by reflecting the caecum medially and dissecting
in its mesentery, and using this route for the revascularization procedure.

The common iliac arteries are cleared and controlled with snares and
atraumatic clamps in order to prevent dislodgment of thrombus into the
legs. The ileocolic artery is then dissected up until a reasonable diameter
(3–4 mm) has been attained, and is controlled with tapes. The vessel is
easily found in the caecal mesentery, and is usually of quite adequate
calibre. A 1 cm arteriotomy is then made in this vessel, and a size 4F
Fogarty embolectomy catheter passed up into the origin of the superior
mesenteric artery (Fig. 5.7). It is gently but persistently worked into the
aorta, if necessary using three or four passages, and repeatedly drawn back
so as to retrieve as much occlusive material as possible. As the occlusion
is extracted, the ileocolic artery progressively dilates. When all possible
thrombus has been withdrawn, the mesentery is milked back to clear the
distal vessels, the SMA flushed from the aorta (Figs. 5.8) and the catheter

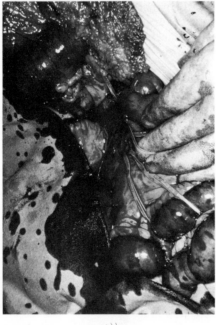

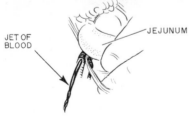

Fig. 5.8. Steps in mesenteric embolectomy: (3) catheter withdrawn—flow re-established.
(Photograph by courtesy of Mr R. W. Marcuson.)

passed again. The iliac arteries are checked, and if any debris is felt to have accumulated within them, this is removed through short longitudinal incisions.

If at this point the SMA picks up pulsation and the bowel becomes pink and is obviously revascularized, the incision in the ileocolic artery is closed, or (if the pattern of collateral appears to make this safe) the vessel is simply ligated. If, however (as is frequently the case), there is still some doubt regarding restoration of blood supply and it is felt that the occlusion at the origin has not been completely relieved, then the bowel must be revascularized in another way. It is quite a simple matter to make a short (1·5 cm) arteriotomy in the right common iliac artery and to carry out a side-to-side anastomosis between this vessel and the already opened ileocolic, using two running sutures of oooo or ooooo material. When clamps are finally removed, the bowel is revascularized in a retrograde fashion, the blood passing up the ileocolic artery into the SMA and hence to the arcades.

Having secured haemostasis and checked the swab count, the abdomen is closed rapidly with one layer of through-and through Nylon sutures

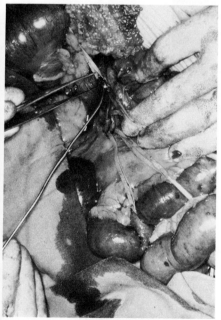

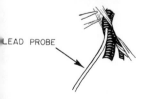

Fig. 5.9 Steps in mesenteric embolectomy: (4) probe introduced into aorta. (Photograph by courtesy of Mr R. W. Marcuson.)

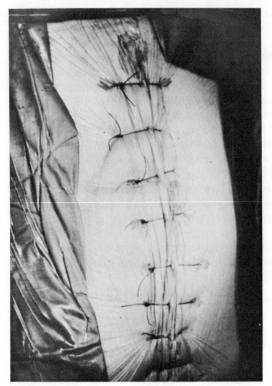

Fig. 5.10. Steps in mesenteric embolectomy: (5) loose closure of the abdomen. (By courtesy of Mr R. W. Marcuson.)

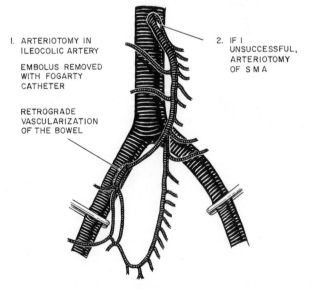

1. ARTERIOTOMY IN
   ILEOCOLIC ARTERY

   EMBOLUS REMOVED
   WITH FOGARTY
   CATHETER

   RETROGRADE
   VASCULARIZATION
   OF THE BOWEL

2. IF I
   UNSUCCESSFUL,
   ARTERIOTOMY
   OF S M A

Fig. 5.11. Alternative technique in mesenteric embolectomy.

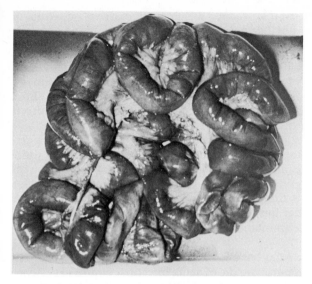

Fig. 5.12. Necrosis of the entire midgut following an apparently successful embolectomy.

(see Fig. 5.10), and the patient returned to the intensive care unit. As has been alluded to before, the practice suggested by Shaw[123, 124] of a routine 'second look' 24 hours later has much to recommend it.

Figure 5.12 illustrates the condition of the intestine 24 hours after what was apparently a successful mesenteric embolectomy with revascularization of the bowel. Clearly, this situation demanded a massive intestinal resection, amounting almost to a complete enterectomy. This produces malabsorption and all the ethical problems associated with maintenance of intravenous nutrition in the 'short bowel syndrome'. Complex as they are, discussion of these problems lies outside the scope of the present work.

The aftermath of revascularization

Depending on the length of time for which the bowel was ischaemic, a period of dysfunction may be expected postoperatively.[46] This was first documented by Shaw and Maynard[124] and by Joske *et al.*[69] who studied the absorptive and exorptive capacities of two patients who had undergone successful relief of thrombosis of the SMA. The subject has been well reviewed by Dardik.[30]

Results of treatment

It must be conceded that the results of treatment of diagnosed intestinal failure are dismally bad. Success is virtually confined to those cases where there is a definite vascular occlusion, and there is only one recorded case in the world literature of a fully documented non-occlusive infarction having survived with treatment.[22] The reasons for this apparently enormous mortality will be apparent from Fig. 4.8, which illustrates the inextricably complicated physiological disturbance which acute massive ischaemia of the midgut engenders. Furthermore, the following factors must be borne in mind:

1. The condition usually occurs in elderly patients, who already have established degenerative disease of the myocardium, lungs and kidneys. It is frequently a complication of central or peripheral circulatory failure, and is an agonal event. Under these circumstances, intestinal failure is more a mode of dying than a cause of death.

2. Much of the study of intestinal failure has been made in the post-mortem room. The autopsy reveals a massive infarction which was quite unsuspected during life, and the pathologist then extrapolates backwards to the clinical events leading up to it.[87] This high preponderance of autopsy studies naturally skews the reported mortality figures. Common sense would suggest that milder forms of the illness occur, which pass unrecognized and either resolve spontaneously or else respond to incidental supportive measures.[112]

3. Almost all authors who have looked at the problem are agreed that a high proportion of patients who die of acute intestinal failure experience a prodrome of abdominal pain, more or less typical of 'intestinal angina' (see Chapter 6). It follows that the factor most likely to improve our mortality figures would be the discovery of a laboratory test which correlates with functionally significant chronic intestinal ischaemia. Although several groups are currently studying this problem, the arrival of such a test is not at present within sight.

References

1   Aakhus, T. (1966). The value of angiography in superior mesenteric artery embolism. *British Journal of Radiology* **39**: 928–934.

2   Aguillon, A., Quilantan, R. and Torres, J. M. (1963). Embolectomia de la arteria mesenterica superior. *Archivos del Instituto de Cardiologia de Mexico* **35**: 50–59.

3   Allgower, M. (1963). Mesenteric embolectomy. *Helvetica Clinica Acta* **30**: 43.

4   Anthony, P. P. (1970). Gangrene of the small intestine—a complication of argentaffin carcinoma. *British Journal of Surgery* **57**: 118–122.

5   Atwell, R. B. (1961). Superior mesenteric artery embolectomy. *Surgery, Gynecology and Obstetrics* **112**: 257–262.

6   Baue, A. E. and Austen, G. W. (1963). Superior mesenteric artery embolism. *Surgery, Gynecology and Obstetrics* **116**: 474–477.

7   Bergan, J. J., Haid, S. P. and Conn, J. (1969). The systemic effects of intestinal revascularization. *American Journal of Surgery* **117**: 235–241.

8   Bergan, J. J., Dry, L., Conn, J. and Trippel, O. H. (1969). Intestinal ischemic syndromes. *Annals of Surgery* **169**: 120–126.

9   Berger, R. L. and Byrne, J. J. (1961). Intestinal gangrene associated with heart disease. *Surgery, Gynecology and Obstetrics* **112**: 529–535.

10 Berry, F. B. and Bougas, J. A. (1950). Agnogenic venous infarction. *Annals of Surgery* **132**: 450–454.

11 Berry, C. L. and Fraser, G. C. (1968). The experimental production of colitis in the rabbit with particular reference to Hirschsprung's disease. *Journal of Pediatric Surgery* **3**: 36–42.

12 Bhagwat, A. G. and Hawk, W. A. (1966). Terminal hemorrhagic necrosing enteropathy (THNE). *American Journal of Gastroenterology* **45**: 163–188.

13 Bigot, J. M., Monnier, J. P., Chermet, J., Kieny, R., Cinqualbre, J. and Tongio, J. (1976) Les ischémies mésentériques aiguës. *Annales de Radiologie* **19**, 377–385.

14 Blennerhasset, J. B. and Reid, J. D. (1960). Intestinal infarction: with particular reference to cases occurring without macroscopic occlusion of vessels. *New Zealand Medical Journal* **59**: 131–138.

15 Bohn, G. L. and Carroll, K. J. (1964). Superior mesenteric embolectomy. *Gut* **5**: 363–364.

16 Bounous, G. (1969). Tryptic enteritis, its role in the pathogenesis of stress ulcer and shock. *Canadian Journal of Surgery* **12**: 397–402.

17 Bowen, A. and Felger, L. (1942). Mesenteric vascular occlusion. *Mississippi Valley Medical Journal* **64**: 24–36.

18 Brawley, R. K., Roberts, W. C. and Morrow, A. G. (1966). Intestinal infarction resulting from nonobstructive mesenteric arterial insufficiency. *Archives of Surgery* **92**: 375–378.

19 Britt, L. G. and Cheek, R. C. (1969). Nonocclusive mesenteric vascular disease. *Annals of Surgery* **169**: 704–711.

20 Brittain, R. S. and Early, T. K. (1963). Emergency thromboendarterectomy of the superior mesenteric artery. *Annals of Surgery* **158**: 138–143.

21 Brooks, D. H. and Bron, K. M. (1975). Postprandial rest-pain and claudication of the lower extremity: a case report. *Surgery* **78**: 677–681.

22 Carey, J. S., Okada, F., Monson, D. O., Yao, S. T. and Shoemaker, W. C. (1967). Intestinal infarction in shock with survival after resection. *Journal of the American Medical Association* **199**: 422–425.

23 Carter, R., Vannis, R., Hinshaw, D. B. and Stafford, C. E. (1959). Inferior mesenteric vascular occlusion—sigmoidoscopic diagnosis. *Surgery* **46**: 845–847.

24 Carter, R., Vannis, R., Hinshaw, D. B. and Stafford, C. E. (1959). Acute inferior mesenteric vascular occlusion—a surgical syndrome. *American Journal of Surgery* **98**: 271–275.

25 Carucci, J. J. (1953). Mesenteric vascular occlusion. *American Journal of Surgery* **85**: 47–51.

26 Castelli, M. F., Qizilbach, A. H., Salem, S. and Fyshe, T. G. (1974). Ischemic bowel disease. *Canadian Medical Association Journal* **111**: 935–941.

27 Chalnot, P., Lochard, J., Frisch, R. and Garolus, J. M. (1962). L'Embolectomie Mésentérique. *Annales de Chirurgie* **16**: 19–24.

27A Chiu, C. J., McArdle, A. H., Brown, R. and Scott, H. J. (1970). Intestinal mucosal lesion in low-flow states. *Archives of Surgery* **101**: 478–483.

28 Connolly, J. E. and Stemmer, E. A. (1973). Intestinal gangrene as the result of mesenteric arterial steal. *American Journal of Surgery* **126**: 197–204.

29 Corday, E. and Williams, J. H. (1960). Effect of shock and vasopressor drugs on brain, heart, kidney and liver. *American Journal of Medicine* **29**: 228–232.

30 Dardik, H. (1970). Intestinal absorption in experimental and clinical mesenteric ischemia. In: *Vascular Disorders of the Intestine*, pp. 531–541. Ed. by S. J. Boley. New York and London, Appleton-Century-Crofts.

31 Demos, N. J., Bahuth, J. J. and Urnes, P. D. (1962). Comparative study of arteriosclerosis in the inferior and superior mesenteric arteries. *Annals of Surgery* **155**: 599–605.

32 de Nord, R. N. and Ring, W. T. (1961). Successful superior mesenteric embolectomy. *Virginia Medical Monthly* **58**: 524–526.

33 Derrick, J. R. and Logan, W. D. (1958). Mesenteric arterial insufficiency. *Surgery* **44**: 823–827.

34 Drucker, W. R., Davis, J. H., Holden, W. D. and Regan, J. R. (1964). Hemorrhagic necrosis of the intestine. *Archives of Surgery* **89**: 42–53.

35 Dumont, A. E., Tice, D. A. and Mulholland, J. M. (1961). Arteriosclerotic occlusion of the superior mesenteric artery. *Annals of Surgery* **154**: 833–838.

36 Dunphy, J. E. (1936). Abdominal pain of vascular origin. *American Journal of Medical Science* **192**: 109–112.

37 Ende, N. P. (1959). Infarction of the bowel in cardiac failure. *New England Journal of Medicine* **260**: 258–851.

38 Fether, J. B. (1959). Gas gangrene as a complication of haematemesis. *British Journal of Surgery* **47**: 187–188.

39 Fick, K. A. and Wolken, A. P. (1949). Necrotic jejunitis. *Lancet* **1**: 519–521.

40 Fine, J. (1958). The role of the intestine in traumatic shock. *American Journal of Gastroenterology* **29**: 596–597.

41 Fogarty, T. J. and Fletcher, W. S. (1966). Genesis of nonocclusive mesenteric ischemia. *American Journal of Surgery* **111**: 130–137.

42 Frengley, J. D. and Reid, J. D. (1964). Nonspecific enteritis resulting from mesenteric vascular insufficiency. *New Zealand Medical Journal* **63**: 212–218.

43 Frimann-Dahl, J. (1960). *Roentgen Examinations in Acute Abdominal* 2nd edn., pp. 324–328. Oxford, Blackwell.

44 Gazes, P. C., Holmes, C. R., Moseley, V. and Pratt-Thomas, H. R. (1961). Acute Hemorrhage and necrosis of the intestines associated with digitalization. *Circulation* **23**: 358–364.

45 Glotzer, D. J. and Shaw, R. S. (1959). Massive bowel infarction. An autopsy study assessing the potentialities of reconstructive vascular surgery. *New England Journal of Medicine* **260**: 162–164.

46 Glotzer, D. J. and Glotzer, P. (1966). Superior mesenteric embolectomy. *Archives of Surgery* **95**: 421–425.

47 Goldgraber, M. B. and Kirsner, J. B. (1959). The Arthus phenomen in the colon of rabbits. *Archives of Pathology* **67**: 556–571.

48 Gooding, R. A. and Couch, R. D. (1962). Mesenteric ischemia without vascular occlusion. *Archives of Surgery* **85**: 186–191.

49 Gordin, R. and Laurent, L. E. (1956). Mesenteric thrombosis and embolism—report of 47 cases. *Acta Medica Scandinavica* **154**: 267–272.

50 Grégoire, R. and Couvelaire, R. (1937). *Apoplexies Viscérales, Sereuses et Hémorrhagiques*. Paris, Masson et Cie.

51 Griessmann, H. (1950). Uber der Darmbrand. *Archiv für Klinische Chirurgie* **1**: 235–240.

52 Grosh, J. L., Mann, R. H. and O'Donnell, W. M. (1965). Nonthrombotic intestinal infarction in heart disease. *American Journal of Medical Sciences* **250**: 613–620.

53 Habbouche, F., Wallace, H. W., Nusbaum, M., Baum, S., Dratch, P. and Blakemore, W. S. (1974). Nonocclusive mesenteric vascular insufficiency. *Annals of Surgery* **180**: 819–822.

54 Haglund, U., Hultén, L., Aksen, C. and Lundgren, O. (1976). Mucosal lesions in the human small intestine in shock. *Gut* **16**: 979–984.

55 Hardy, E. G. (1963). Superior mesenteric embolectomy. *British Medical Journal* **1**: 1658.

56 Harris, P. L. and Charlesworth, D. (1974). Chronic intestinal ischaemia due to aorto-iliac steal. *Journal of Cardiovascular Surgery* **15**: 122–124.

57 Heer, F. W., Silen, W. and French, S. W. (1965). Intestinal gangrene without apparent vascular occlusion. *American Journal of Surgery* **110**: 231–238.

58 Hendry, W. G. (1948). Occlusion of the superior mesenteric artery. *British Medical Journal* **1**: 144.

59 Hoffman, F. S., Zimmerman, S. K. and Cardwell, E. S. (1960). Massive intestinal infarction without vascular occlusion associated with aortic insufficiency. *New England Journal of Medicine* **263**: 436–440.

60 Holle, F., Schutz, R. and Becker, F. (1958). Enterocolitis Acute Pseudomembranacea: eine Postoperativ Zweiterkrankus. *Archiv für Klinische Chirurgie* **288**: 219.

61 Hostetler, T. G., Lewis, H. D. and Hayes, W. L. (1965). Heart failure simulating an acute surgical abdomen. *American Journal of Cardiology* **16**: 576–579.

62 Hurwitz, A. and Khalif, R. A. (1960). Acute necrotizing enterocolitis proximal to obstructing neoplasms of the colon. *Surgery, Gynecology and Obstetrics* **111**: 749–752.

63 Irving, D. W. and Corday, E. (1961). Effect of cardiac arrhythmias on the renal and mesenteric circulation. *American Journal of Cardiology* **8**: 32.

64 Jago, R. H. (1971). Superior mesenteric embolectomy. *British Journal of Surgery* **58**: 628–631.

65 Jenson, C. B. and Smith, G. A. (1956). A clinical study of 51 cases of mesenteric infarction. *Surgery* **40**: 930–937.

66 Johnson, C. C. and Baggenstoss, A. H. (1949). Mesenteric vascular occlusion. *Proceedings of the Staff Meeting of the Mayo Clinic* **24**: 649–653.

67 Johnson, W. C. and Nabseth, D. C. (1974). Visceral infarction following aortic surgery. *Annals of Surgery* **180**: 312–318.

68 Jordan, P. H., Boulafendis, D. and Guinn, G. A. (1970). Factors other than major vascular occlusion that contribute to intestinal infarction. *Annals of Surgery* **171**: 189–192.

69 Joske, R. A., Shamma'a, M. H. and Drummey, G. D. (1958). Intestinal malabsorption following temporary occlusion of the superior mesenteric artery. *American Journal of Medicine* **25**: 449–457.

70 Katz, A. M. (1959). Hemorrhagic duodenitis in myocardial infarction. *Annals of Intestinal Medicine* **51**: 212–214.

71 Kay, A. W., Richards, R. L. and Watson, A. J. (1958). Acute necrotizing (pseudomembranous) enterocolitis. *British Journal of Surgery* **46**: 45.

72 Kieny, R., Cinqualbre, J., Pinke, R. and Jeanblanc, B. (1974). Chirurgie des lésions athéromateuses des artères digestives. In: *Chirurgie des Arteriopathies Digestives*, pp. 141–148. Paris, Expansion Scientifique.

73 Killingback, M. J. and Lloyd Williams, K. W. (1962). Necrotizing colitis. *British Journal of Surgery* **49**: 175–185.

74 Klass, A. A. (1951). Embolectomy in acute mesenteric occlusion. *Annals of Surgery* **134**: 913–917.

75 Kleckner, M. S., Bargen, J. A. and Baggenstoss, A. H. (1952). Pseudomembranous enterocolitis. *Gastroenterology* **21**: 212–216.

76 Kleitsch, W. P., Connors, E. K. and O'Neill, T. J. (1957). Surgical operations on the superior mesenteric artery. *Archives of Surgery* **75**: 752–760.

77 Klemperer, P., Penner, A. and Bernheim, A. I. (1946). The gastrointestinal manifestations of shock. *American Journal of Digestive Diseases* **7**: 410–415.

78 Kligerman, M. J. and Vidone, R. A. (1965). Intestinal infarction in the absence of occlusive mesenteric vascular disease. *American Journal of Cardiology* **16**: 562–570.

79 Kodsi, B. E. (1969). Probable extensive ischemic damage of the small bowel with spontaneous recovery. *New England Journal of Medicine* **281**: 309.

80 Kountz, S. L., Lamb, D. R. and Connolly, J. E. (1966). Aortoiliac Steal Syndrome. *Archives of Surgery* **92**: 490–494.

81 Lancaster, J. R., Payan, H. M., Jacobs, W. H. and Gerwig, W. H. (1967). Aortoiliac steal syndrome and necrosis of gastrointestinal tract. *Archives of Surgery* **94**: 172–174.

81A   Kreager, J. A., Wheat, M. W., Weigel, W. W. and Cievasse, L. (1965). Superior mesenteric artery embolectomy. *American Surgeon* **31**: 116–120.

82   Lefer, A. M. (1970). Role of a myocardial depressant factor in the pathogenesis of circulatory shock. *Federation Proceedings* **29**: 1836–1847.

83   Levine, S. (1959). Intestinal infarction without vascular occlusion. *American Journal of Proctology* **10**: 257–263.

84   Liavåg, I. (1967). Acute mesenteric vascular insufficiency. *Acta Chirurgica Scandinavica* **133**: 631–639.

85   Lillehei, R. C. (1957). The intestinal factor in irreversible hemorrhagic shock. *Surgery* **42**: 1043–1059.

86   Lillehei, R. C., Longerbeam, J. K., Bloch, J. H. and Manax, W. G. (1964). The nature of irreversible shock. *Annals of Surgery* **160**: 682–710.

87   McGovern, V. J. and Goulstone, S. G. M. (1965). Ischaemic enterocolitis. *Gut* **6**: 213–220.

88   MacGregor, A. M. C., Abney, H. T. and Morris, L. (1974). Pharmacodynamic response in non-occlusive mesenteric ischemia. *American Surgeon* **40**: 381–383.

89   Mackenzie, R. L. and Provan, J. L. (1974). Recognition and management of embolism to the superior mesenteric artery. *Canadian Medical Association Journal* **111**, 1207–1210.

90   MacMahon, H. E. (1972). Systemic scleroderma and massive infarction of intestine and liver. *Surgery, Gynecology and Obstetrics* **134**: 10–14.

91   Marston, A. (1962). The bowel in shock. *Lancet* **2**: 365–370.

92   Marston, A. (1963). Causes of death in mesenteric arterial occlusion: 1. Local and general effects of devascularization of the bowel. 2. Observations on revascularization of the ischemic bowel. *Annals of Surgery* **158**: 952–969.

93   Marston, A., Marcuson, R. W., Chapman, M. and Arthur, J. F. (1969). Experimental study of devascularization of the colon. *Gut* **10**: 121–130.

94   Marston, A., Szilagyi, D. E., Kieny, R. and Taylor, G. W. (1976). Intestinal ischemia. *Archives of Surgery* **111**: 107–112.

95   Martinis, A., Crystal, D. K., Wagner, C. L., Cobb, A. W. and Day, S. W. (1962). Superior mesenteric artery occlusion. *Western Journal of Surgery* **70**: 6–8.

96   Mavor, G. E., Lyall, A. D., Chrystal, K. M. R. and Tsapogas, M. (1962). Mesenteric infarction as a vascular emergency. *British Journal of Surgery* **50**: 219–222.

97   Miller, H. I. and di Mare, S. A. (1958). Report of a case of superior mesenteric embolectomy and small bowel resection with recovery. *New England Journal of Medicine* **259**: 512–513.

98   Ming, S. C. and Levitan, R. (1960). Acute hemorrhagic necrosis of the gastrointestinal tract. *New England Journal of Medicine* **263**: 59–63.

99   Murrell, T. G. C. and Roth, L. (1963). Necrotizing jejunitis: a newly discovered disease in the highlands of New Guinea. *Medical Journal of Australia* **1**: 61–69.

100   Murrell, T.G. C., Roth, L., Egerton, J., Samels, J. and Walker, P. D. (1966). Pig-bel: enteritis necroticans. *Lancet* **1**: 217–222.

101   Musa, B. U. (1965). Intestinal infarction without mesenteric vascular occlusion. *Annals of Internal Medicine* **63**: 783–792.

102   Olsen, V. B. and Sauter, K. E. (1965). Superior mesenteric embolectomy. *Angiology* **16**: 121–129.

103   Orr, T. G., Lorhan, P. H. and Kaul, P. G. (1954). Mesenteric vascular occlusion. *Journal of the American Medical Association* **155**: 648–651.

104   Ottinger, L. W. and Austen, W. G. (1967). A study of 136 patients with mesenteric infarction. *Surgery, Gynecology and Obstetrics* **124**: 251–261.

105 Ottinger, L. W. (1974). Nonocclusive mesenteric infarction. *Surgical Clinics of North America* **54**: 689–698.

106 Patterson, M. and Rosenbaum, H. D. (1952). Enteritis necroticans. *Gastroenterology* **21**: 110–116.

107 Pawlik, W. and Jacobson, E. D. (1974). Effects of digoxin on the mesenteric circulation. *Cardiovascular Research Center Bulletin* **12**: 80–84.

108 Penn, I. (1970). Major colonic problems in human homotransplant recipients. (1970). *Archives of Surgery* **100**: 61–65.

109 Penner, A. and Bernheim, A. I. (1939). Acute postoperative enterocolitis—a study on the pathologic nature of shock. *Archives of Pathology* **27**: 966–971.

110 Perloff, L. J., Chou, H., Petrella, E. J., Grossman, R. A. and Barker, C. F. (1976). Acute colitis in the renal allograft recipient. *Annals of Surgery* **183**: 77–83.

111 Polansky, B. J., Berger, R. L. and Byrne, J. J. (1964). Massive non-occlusive intestinal infarction associated with digitalis toxicity. *Circulation* (supplement) **30**: 141–145.

112 Pope, C. H. and O'Neal, R. M. (1956). Incomplete infarction of ileum simulating regional enteritis. *Journal of the American Medical Association* **161**: 963–964.

113 Powis, S. J. A., Barnes, A. D., Dawson-Edwards, P. and Thompson, R. (1972). Ileocolonic problems after cadaveric renal transplantation. *British Medical Journal* **1**: 99–101.

114 Prandi, D., Degott, C., Molas, G. and Lortat-Jacob, I.-L. (1975). Entérites et colites ischémiques aigues post-opératoires. *Archives Francaises des Maladies de l'Appareil Digestif* **64**: 209–214.

115 Reivich, M. A., Holling, H. E., Roberts, B. and Toole, J. F. (1961). Reversal of blood-flow through the vertebral artery and its effect on the cerebral circulation. *New England Journal of Medicine* **265**: 868–872.

116 Renton, C. J. C. (1972). Non-occlusive intestinal infarction. *Clinics in Gastroenterology* **1**: 655–671.

117 Renwick, S. B., McGovern, V. J. and Spence, J. (1966). Necrotizing enterocolitis. *Medical Journal of Australia* **2**: 413–416.

118 Saris, D. S. and Uricchio, J. F. (1960). Superior mesenteric arterial embolectomy. *Archives of Surgery* **81**: 90–95.

119 Sasser, C., Farringer, J. L. and Pickens, D. R. (1971). Superior mesenteric embolectomy. *American Surgeon* **37**: 319–322.

120 Schoofs, E., Vereecken, L. and Derom, F. (1975). Acute occlusie van der arteria mesenterica superior. *Acta Chirurgica Belgica* **74**: 86–92.

121 Senn, A., Gradel, F., Lundsgaard Hansen, P. and Wälti, R. (1961). Die operative Behandlung der Peripheren und Mesenterialen Embolie. *Schweize Medizinische Wochenschrift* **91**: 525–533.

122 Sharefkin, J. B. and Silen, W. (1974). Diuretic agents. Inciting factors in nonocclusive mesenteric infarction? *Journal of the American Medical Association* **229**: 1451–1453.

123 Shaw, R. S. and Rutledge, R. H. (1957). Superior mesenteric embolectomy in the treatment of massive mesenteric infarction. *New England Journal of Medicine* **257**: 595–600.

124 Shaw, R. S. and Maynard, E. P. (1958). Acute and chronic thrombosis of the mesenteric arteries associated with malabsorption. *New England Journal of Medicine* **258**: 874–878.

125 Skinner, D. B., Zarins, C. and Moossa, A. R. (1974). Mesenteric vascular disease. *American Journal of Surgery* **128**: 835–839.

126 Sorensen, F. H. and Vetner, M. (1969). Haemorrhagic mucosal necrosis of

the gastrointestinal tract without vascular occlusion. *Acta Chirurgica Scandinavica* **135**: 439–448.

127 Stewart, G. D., Sweetman, W. R., Westphal, K. and Wise, R. A. (1960). Superior mesenteric artery embolectomy. *Annals of Surgery* **151**: 274–280.

128 Stewart, J. O. R. (1963). Portal gas embolism, a prognostic sign in mesenteric vascular occlusion. *British Medical Journal* **1**: 1328.

129 Strandness, D. E. and Sumner, D. S. Aorto-iliac steal. In: *Hemodynamics for Surgeons*, pp. 376–380. New York, Grune & Stratton (1975).

130 Todd, I. A. D. and Pearson, F. G. (1963). Mesenteric vascular occlusion. Analysis of a series of cases and report of a successful embolectomy. *Canadian Journal of Surgery* **6**: 33–35.

131 Vyden, J. K. (1972). The systemic effects of acute superior mesenteric vascular insufficiency. In: *Vascular Disorders of the Intestine*, pp. 279–294. Ed. by S. J. Boley. New York and London. Appleton-Century-Crofts.

131A Wangensteen, S. L., Golden, G. T. and Stapleton, S. L. (1972). Successsful superior mesenteric artery embolectomy. *American Journal of Surgery* **123**: 601–603.

132 Whitehead, R. (1971). Ischaemic enterocolitis, an expression of the intravascular coagulation syndrome. *Gut* **12**: 912–917.

133 Whitehead, R. The pathology of intestinal ischaemia. *Clinics in Gastroenterology* **1**: 613–637.

134 Wiggers, C. J. (1943) Splanchnic pooling in haemorrhagic shock. *Journal of Experimental Medicine and Surgery* **1**: 2–10.

135 Williams, L. F., Anastasia, L. F., Hasiokis, C. A., Bosniak, M. A. and Byrne, J. J. (1967). Non-occlusive mesenteric infarction. *American Journal of Surgery* **114**: 374–381.

136 Williams, L. F., Kim, R. M., Tompkins, W. and Byrne, J. J. (1968). Aortoiliac steal—a cause of intestinal ischaemia. *New England Journal of Medicine* **278**: 777–778.

137 Wilson, R. and Qualheim, R. E. (1954). A form of acute hemorrhagic enterocolitis afflicting chronically ill individuals. *Gastroenterology* **27**: 431–436.

138 Zeissler, J. and Rassfeld-Sternberg, L. (1949). Necrotizing jejunitis. *British Medical Journal* **1**: 267–269.

139 Zimmerman, H. J. and West, M. (1964). Serum enzyme changes in intestinal ischemia. *Medical Clinics of North America* **48**: 189–195.

140 Zuidema, G. D. (1961). Surgical management of superior mesenteric arterial emboli. *Archives of Surgery* **82**: 267–276.

141 Zuidema, G. D., Reed, P., Turcotte, J. and Fry, W. J. (1964). Superior mesenteric embolectomy. *Annals of Surgery* **159**: 158–162.

6

Chronic Intestinal Ischaemia

Introduction

The concept of intestinal pain originating from chronic arterial obstruction, analogous to angina pectoris or to calf claudication, is appealing in its simplicity, and has been mentioned in medical writing since the beginning of this century.[61, 77] Various names have been given to it, such as 'abdominal claudication', 'abdominal angina' and 'mesenteric angina' and these have been criticized on various grounds. For instance, 'claudication' refers strictly to a disturbance of gait, 'abdominal angina' has been used to describe myocardial pain referred to the abdomen, and it is the intestine rather than the mesentery which is the ischaemic organ. The subject was reviewed by Mikkelsen,[62] who put forward the term 'intestinal angina', the general adoption of which was later advocated and is now generally accepted.

Until the middle years of the twentieth century, when it became possible for the radiologist to visualize, and for the surgeon to reconstruct, the aorta and its branches, the concept of intestinal angina remained largely academic. However, interest was generated by Dunphy's[23] demonstration that of 12 patients dying from mesenteric thrombosis, 7 gave a prodromal history of a quite characteristic abdominal pain, occurring in close relation to meals. He showed that this prodromal period was usually short, never exceeding two years, and suggested that if such patients could be identified early in the course of their disease then not only might their pain be relieved, but perhaps also the lethal infarction could be avoided by a timely arterial reconstruction.

It has been known for a long time that whereas acute occlusion of the SMA is almost always fatal, a block which builds up slowly enough for collateral circulation to develop may be quite well tolerated, and indeed may cause no symptoms. There was, for instance, the famous case of the body received for dissection at the Edinburgh Medical School in 1868, which was reported by Chiene.[10] The body was that of a 65-year-old woman who had died of 'paralysis' and was not known to have had any abdominal symptoms during life. She was found to have an aortic aneurysm, with complete obliteration of both coeliac axis and SMA. The bowel was nourished by extracoelomic vessels and by the superior haemorrhoidal artery, which was enlarged to the size of the femoral. Since that date, many other cases of chronic occlusion of the visceral arteries have been reported and treated, with varying success (see Table 6.1). The incidence and distribution of occlusion in the visceral arteries have been established by studies of autopsy material carried out by Maljatzkaja,[52]

Johnson,[41] Carucci,[9] Derrick[18] and Reiner.[70] These authors all reached very similar conclusions, which can be summarized as follows:

1. Atheroma of the visceral arteries is common, and increases with age, although it may begin during the second and third decades. Between one-third and one-half of all subjects over the age of 45 show some narrowing of the coeliac axis and/orSMA. Where arteriosclerotic changes are present elsewhere in the body, the figure rises to between one-half and three-quarters.

2. The coeliac axis and SMA are affected in roughly equal proportions, the IMA rather less so.

3. Lesions are mainly confined to the aortic origin of the vessels. It is unusual to find stenoses or atheromatous plaques in the individual intestinal arteries.

4. The gross appearance of the bowel is the same, whether or not such arterial lesions are present.

We are here confronted with a difficulty, which simply stated is this:

Stenoses and occlusions of the visceral arteries are common lesions, as demonstrated on angiograms or at post-mortem, but intestinal angina is an extremely rare symptom. It is, none the less one which is important to identify, not only because of the severe distress which it causes, but also because it implies a direct threat to life. A test designed to pick out the type of arterial occlusion which poses such a threat is badly needed but is at present not available.

The diagnosis of obscure abdominal pain forms a major part of every clinician's daily work. The patient presents with chronic distressing symptoms but without corroborative physical signs, and simple conventional diagnostic methods fail to reveal an anatomical fault. This situation is particularly common in the middle-aged and elderly, who are at the same time prone to various types of cardiovascular illness. To assign their symptoms to vascular disease of the alimentary tract is a convenient short cut to accurate diagnostic thinking, but may at the same time carry considerable danger to the patient, who may be subjected to intensive investigation and even perhaps an ambitious but inappropriate surgical operation. It is the purpose of this chapter to examine critically the concept of chronic intestinal ischaemia, and to consider what it has to offer to the patient, and to the doctor, in practical terms.

The clinical picture of intestinal angina

Symptoms

As classically described, the patient with one or more occluded visceral arteries complains of cramping abdominal pain occurring in very strict relationship to meals, and usually between 20 and 50 minutes after ingestion of food. The pain is centred on the epigastrium but radiates all over the abdomen, and is of a cramping colicky nature. It is on occasions relieved by standard analgesic agents, and by 'vasodilator' drugs. As the disease progresses, the pain becomes so severe that the patient becomes terrified of eating (the classical symptom of 'food fear') and loss of weight inevitably follows. Reluctance to eat is quite enough to explain the observed weight loss, which is almost certainly due to diminished intake rather than to interference with absorption.

Together with the pain and weight loss, there is a disturbance in bowel habit. Most authors report initial constipation, due to diminished bulk intake, which is later followed by diarrhoea secondary to malabsorption of fat. However, study of the literature[4, 5, 16, 17, 28, 36, 43, 47, 48, 53, 57, 58, 81, 90] discloses no very consistent pattern of bowel symptomatology.

Many patients (indeed, perhaps the majority) present as an abdominal emergency, as an incidental crisis precipitates their chronic intestinal ischaemia into acute intestinal failure. In these cases, the prodromal syndrome of pain, loss of weight and disturbance of bowel habit will often have been dismissed as a neurotic complaint, or misinterpreted as terminal malignant disease. Associated disease in other parts of the cardiovascular system is the rule. By this is meant a past history of myocardial infarct, episodes of left ventricular failure, arterial hypertension and chronic renal failure, and occlusive disease of the aortofemoral segment resulting in ischaemic pain in the lower limbs.

Physical signs

The patient is described as presenting a picture of emaciated misery, with the scars of several previous ineffective abdominal operations.

The physical sign which is most constantly referred to in the medical literature is the finding of a loud systolic bruit in the upper abdomen, midway between the umbilicus and xiphisternum, and corresponding to the position of the superior mesenteric artery. This was found, for instance, in 21 out of the 24 patients reported by Reul *et al.*[71] However, this physical sign is of (to say the least) doubtful validity. Not only is such a bruit a frequent accompaniment of atheromatous roughening of the aorta (which is almost invariably found in this age group), but recent studies[25, 42] have demonstrated that it can be heard in a large proportion of asymptomatic young men and women. The other physical sign which has been mentioned is the finding of exaggerated bowel sounds following meals. Once again, however, this is clearly a highly subjective finding which is difficult to confirm or reproduce.

Radiological appearances

In practice, the diagnosis is made by exclusion. That is to say, the patient presents with a non-specific picture of obscure abdominal pain and weight loss, and is then subjected to the normal gamut of examination designed to exclude organic disease of the upper gastrointestinal tract. These will include barium studies, fibrendoscopy of stomach, duodenum and colon, with screening of the oesophagus and gravitational search for reflux, and gastric and small bowel studies to exclude peptic ulceration and inflammatory bowel disease. Additionally, an oral cholecystogram will have been carried out with negative results, and most patients will have had an in-

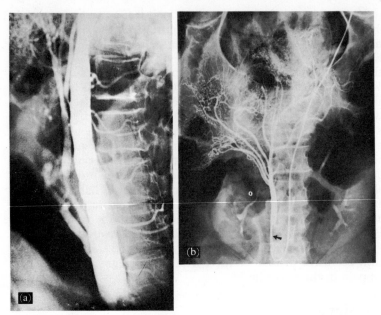

Fig. 6.1 Stenosis of SMA: (a) AP view; (b) lateral view. (Reproduced from Marston, 1972, *Annals of the Royal College of Surgeons*, **50**: 327, by kind permission of the Honorary Editor.)

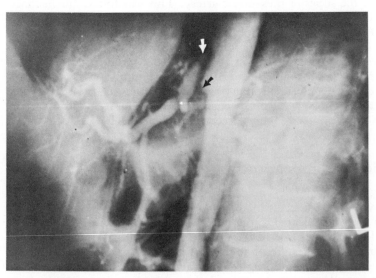

Fig. 6.2 Complete occlusion of SMA, with stenosis of coeliac axis. (Reproduced from Marston, 1972, *Annals of the Royal College of Surgeons*, **50**: 327, by kind permission of the Honorary Editor.)

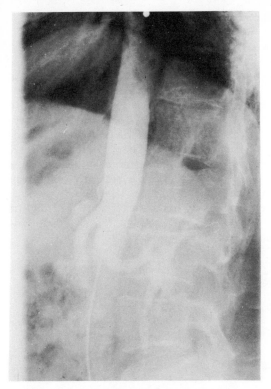

Fig. 6.3. Stenosis of coeliac axis, with normal SMA, in an asymptomatic patient investigated for hypertension.

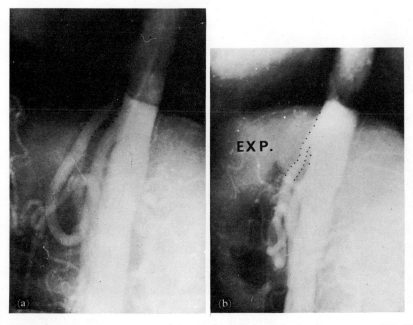

EXP.

(a) (b)

Fig. 6.4. Coeliac axis stenosis: (a) in inspiration; (b) in expiration (by courtesy of Dr Hans Herlinger).

travenous pyelogram. These negative examinations will have prompted the need for aortography.

The diagnosis of intestinal angina depends on the correlation of clinical symptoms with aortographic findings. It is essential to examine the contrast-filled aorta in both anteroposterior and lateral projections, and also to carry out selective examination of the three main visceral trunks. A varying pattern of occlusion, roughly corresponding to the post-mortem findings outlined above, will be demonstrated. These appearances are illustrated in Figs. 6.1–6.6. However, the demonstration of a stenosis on an x-ray film is in fact of little help in explaining a patient's symptoms, and still less in recommending a line of treatment.

As already pointed out, the human body has great capacity for building

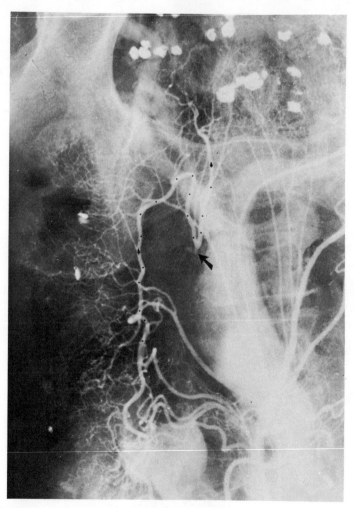

Fig. 6.5. Occlusion of the IMA, showing nourishment of the colon via the marginal artery (by courtesy of Dr Hans Herlinger).

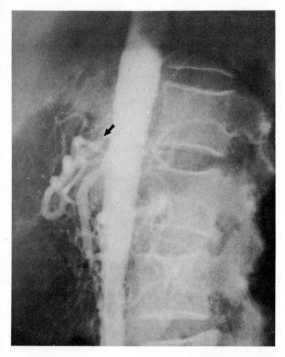

Fig. 6.6. Stenosis of the coeliac axis, with partial occlusion of SMA and total occlusion of IMA. (Reproduced from Marston, 1972, *Annals of the Royal College of Surgeons*, **50**: 327, by kind permission of the Honorary Editor.)

collateral flow around a blocked visceral artery, and the incidence of asymptomatic stenosis is extremely high. Dick *et al.*[20] studied 1,000 aortograms obtained from patients with and without abdominal symptoms, in order to provide some idea of the relationship between blood flow (as estimated by the summed cross-sectional areas of the arteries) and symptomatology. Eleven of their patients had undergone aortography because of suspected intestinal angina and, of these, 6 were found to have other diseases common to this age group. The remaining 5 had variable symptoms which suggested mesenteric vascular disease. Of these 5 patients the fact of chronic intestinal ischaemia was proven in 2, of whom 1 had complete relief of symptoms following arterial reconstruction.

Intestinal function

It seems logical to suppose that reduction in blood supply to the alimentary tract would produce absorptive or exsorptive abnormalities which could be measured in the clinical laboratory. In fact, studies of this nature are not easy to come by, and tend to disagree. Thus while some workers[17, 56, 58, 64] were unable to demonstrate any functional abnormality in intestinal ischaemia, others[83] found steatorrhoea which disappeared following arterial reconstruction. A study by Webb and Hardy[89] demonstrated an abnormal absorption of carbohydrate and fat, measured respectively by the *d*-xylose and ^{131}I triolein techniques, which was corrected by aorto-SMA bypass. Larson[48] reported abnormal serum carotene levels and increase in faecal fat, and Dardik[16] confirmed abnormal preoperative serum carotene values; delayed absorption of radioiodinated triolein, and impaired *d*-xylose absorption in their patient with SMA stenosis, which reverted to normal following operation. Our own experience has concentrated more on the study of protein-losing enteropathy, and we have demonstrated in three patients[56] an abnormal faecal loss of ^{51}Cr-labelled albumin, associated with symptomatic SMA stenosis which was, if not wholly corrected, at any rate redirected towards normal values, following arterial reconstruction.

Delmont,[17] in a study of 15 patients with established occlusive lesions of the coeliac axis and superior mesenteric artery, encountered 1 patient who excreted more than 5 g of fat per day, 3 with more than 10 per cent retention of isotope-labelled vitamin B_{12} (Schilling test), 1 with greater than normal excretion of ^{131}I-labelled PVP and 2 with less than 1·25 g excretion of a 5-g dose of *d*-xylose. All other patients studied were completely normal. There is, in fact, very little evidence of abnormalities of absorptive or exsorptive function arising from stenoses at the origins of the visceral arteries. The subject has been well reviewed by Dardik.[16]

Management of a suspected case of intestinal angina

From what has been said above, it is clear that this syndrome is difficult to define. The symptoms are variable, the physical signs absent or of doubtful significance, the radiological appearances undependable and the laboratory studies unhelpful. None the less, the challenging fact remains that many people do die each year from (possibly) preventable mesenteric infarction, and that a fair proportion describe a prodromal history which, if recognized in time, could lead to appropriate avoiding action. It is therefore important for the clinician to keep in mind the possibility of chronic ischaemia in any case of obscure abdominal pain.

Clearly, the first essential is to eliminate, by ordinary methods of history taking, physical examination, endoscopy, x-ray and laboratory investigation, the common and remediable conditions. It is apparent from the literature of this subject that many patients subjected to aortography because of suspected mesenteric vascular insufficiency in fact should never have been examined in this way, because a subsequent laparotomy has disclosed another, more mundane, disease.[72, 74, 75]

It none the less does happen on occasion that a patient continues to complain of abdominal pain and continues to remain unwell, for reasons which elude conventional investigation and, because of his background, history and age group, the suspicion of intestinal arterial disease becomes stronger. In these circumstances further study is justified. This should include full tests of intestinal absorptive and exsorptive function, including:

Full blood-picture, haemoglobin, indices, serum iron, folate and B_{12} levels

Liver function tests and serum enzymes

Carotene levels

Glucose tolerance test

d-Xylose absorption, 5-day fat balance, Schilling test for B_{12} absorption

Examination of faecal radioactivity following intravenous ^{51}Cr

Fibrendoscopy with direct vision biopsy of several jejunal sites, which are then subjected to conventional light and electron microscopic study

Full biplane aortography with free and selective catheterization of the CA, SMA and IMA

This full evaluation of every case not only helps the individual patient but may perhaps in the future provide us with a working profile of the disease which will enable us to identify others at risk. A corollary of this is that such information should be pooled, so that the contribution of each individual clinician can be added to a common data bank. This, perhaps, is a justification for the list of workers referred to in the Introduction.

Operative techniques

It must be admitted that surgical enthusiasm has, to an extent, outrun science in the management of this condition. There have been many series of operations reported in the literature, designed rather to correct an aortographic appearance than to improve the physiological disturbance (whatever that may be). These are set out in Table 6.1 and are, basically, of two types, namely:

1. Direct attack on the ostial lesion. In the case of the coeliac axis this is the only possible method, due to the configuration of the artery. It may also be used for the SMA, although here there are possible alternative methods.

2. The other method comprises an indirect attack on the mesenteric system, avoiding the difficult territory of the origin of the SMA, and having the advantage that it can be accomplished through a purely abdominal operation.

Exposure of the visceral trunks

All authorities are agreed that this is best and most safely accomplished via a thoracoabdominal incision[38, 48, 84] (see Fig. 6.7). This allows a complete and safe exposure of the supra- and infradiaphragmatic aorta, the median arcuate ligament, the origin of the coeliac axis, the mouth of the SMA, the neck of the pancreas and both renal arteries.

With the patient in an appropriate half-lateral position, the incision is developed along the line of the eighth rib, crosses the costal margin and is prolonged downwards into the left rectus sheath. The muscle layers are divided with diathermy, and the ribs spread apart with a Finochietto type rib spreader. The abdominal contents are then carefully checked over in order to exclude non-vascular pathology. The diaphragm is incised circumferentially, to avoid dividing terminal branches of the phrenic nerve, to an extent which allows complete exposure of the thoracoabdominal cavi-

Table 6.1 Reconstructions of visceral arteries

Reference	Sex and age of patient	Lesion	Operation	Result
Mikkelsen & Zaro, 1959[63]	M/62	SMA stenosis Aortic occlusion	SMA endarterectomy	Well at 40 months
Starzl & Trippel, 1959[85]	M/62	SMA stenosis Aortic occlusion	Endarterectomy of aorta+renal+SMA	Well at 12 months
Derrick et al., 1959[18]	M/67	SMA stenosis	Bypass homograft aorta→CA+SMA	Well at 2 weeks
Mikkelsen & Berne, 1962[64]	M/57	CA occlusion SMA stenosis	CA+SMA endarterectomy	Well at 18 months
Morris et al, 1962[65]	F/48	SMA stenosis Aortoiliac occlusion	Bifurcation prosthesis with side-arm to SMA	Well at 18 months
	M/65	CA stenosis SMA occlusion	Aortosplenic bypass with arm to SMA	Well at 11 months
	F/67	CA stenosis	Aortosplenic prosthesis	Well at 2 years
	F/61	CA+SMA stenosis	Bypass prosthesis aorta→SMA+ splenic artery	Well at 5 months
	M/53	CA+SMA stenosis IMA occlusion	Aortosplenic prosthesis	Well at 3 months
	M/74	CA+SMA+IMA stenosis	Aortic prosthesis→ splenic+SMA	Well at 1 year
	M/63	CA stenosis+IMA occlusion	Aortosplenic prosthesis	Well at 2 months
Webb & Hardy 1962[89]	M/63	SMA occlusion	Aortomesenteric bypass	Well at 15 months
Mavor & Lyall, 1962[60]	M/75	CA+SMA stenosis	Iliomesenteric bypass	
Masson & Staymans 1962[58]	F/65	CA+SMA stenosis	SMA endarterectomy	Well at 3 years
Ranger & Spence, 1962[69]	M	SMA occlusion	Iliomesenteric anastomosis	Well at 3 years

Author	Age/Sex	Diagnosis	Procedure	Outcome
Vollmar et al., 1964[87]	M/52	CA+SMA occlusion	SMA reimplantation	Well at 2 months
	F/63	SMA stenosis	Aortocoeliac prosthesis	Unstated
Dardik et al., 1965[16]	F/70	CA stenosis	Side-arm from aorto-femoral prosthesis to splenic artery+SMA	Well at 5 months
van Zyl & du Toit 1966[91]	M/68	SMA occlusion	Ilioaortic anastomosis	Well at 3 months
Stoney & Wylie, 1966[84]	not given	CA+SMA stenosis +IMA (2)	Endarterectomy (4)	1 death
		CA+SMA stenosis (3) SMA stenosis (1)	Reimplantation (2)	1 occlusion 4 satisfactory
Marston, 1970[56]	F/57	SMA occlusion	Aortomesenteric anastomosis	Well at 5 years
	M/50	CA occlusion SMA stenosis	Patch angioplasty CA	Unchanged at 1 year
	M/66	CA+SMA stenosis	Patch angioplasty CA	Well at 2 years
	M/67	SMA occlusion	Aortomesenteric anastomosis	Well at 3 years
	F/58	CA+SMA occlusion	Aortomesenteric anastomosis	Well at 1 year
	M/70	SMA occlusion	Endarterectomy + aortomesenteric anastomosis	Well at 1 year
Marston, 1976 (unpublished)	M/64	CA+SMA+IMA occlusion	Aorto-SMA anastomosis	Death at 6 weeks from myocardial infarction
	F/48	CA stenosis SMA occlusion IMA occlusion	Aorto-SMA anastomosis	Postoperative death from intestinal infarction
	M/64	CA occlusion SMA stenosis	Patch angioplasty CA	Symptoms persist at 1 year
	F/68	CA stenosis SMA occlusion IMA stenosis	Aorto-SMA Dacron shunt	Well at 1 year
	M/57	CA stenosis SMA occlusion	Aorto-SMA anastomosis	Well at 6 months

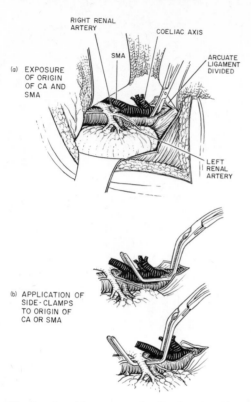

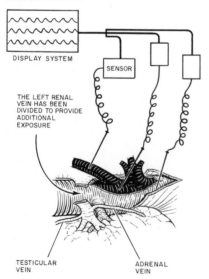

Fig. 6.7. Arterial reconstruction for chronic midgut ischaemia: (a) Exposure; (b) Clamping of CA and SMA.

Fig. 6.8. Arterial reconstruction for chronic midgut ischaemia: division of renal vein and measurement of pressure gradients.

ties. The peritoneum behind the spleen is incised and the spleen, the splenic vessels and the tail of the pancreas are mobilized over to the right, carrying with them the fundus of the stomach, until the aorta is clearly seen. Careful dissection with forward mobilization of the lymph nodes and vessels will expose the origin of the coeliac axis as it emerges from beneath the median arcuate ligament. Keeping close to the wall of the aorta, a plane of dissection can be developed which leads directly downwards to the origin of the SMA (Fig. 6.7a), which usually lies between 1 and 2 cm below that of the coeliac axis. Lateral clearance of the aorta brings into view the origins of the renal arteries, which are identified for their later preservation.

Having inspected and palpated the obstructing lesions, pressure measurements are taken in order to determine whether a significant gradient exists. A needle connected to a standard transducer and display device is inserted into the aorta, the coeliac axis and the superior mesenteric artery, and pressures recorded at a stable state (Fig. 6.8). If an electromagnetic flowmeter is available, it is conveniently applied at this stage.

The exact form of reconstruction will clearly depend on the symptomatology, the aortographic appearances and the recorded pressure and flow profile. Available techniques are as follows:

1. Division of the median arcuate ligament of the diaphragm, freeing the origin of the coeliac axis. This is discussed in detail below.

2. Patch angioplasty of the coeliac axis. This requires application of a side-clamp to the aorta (see Fig. 6.7b) and coeliac axis, followed by a longitudinal incision across the origin of the vessels, and insertion of a patch of Teflon, Dacron or previously removed distal saphenous vein, to broaden the origin.

3. Alternatively, the coeliac axis can be detached and reimplanted, following similar application of a side-clamp to the aorta.

Exactly the same techniques can be applied to the SMA, with the proviso that great care must be taken not to occlude the origins of the renal arteries when the clamp is applied. Following reconstruction, the pressure gradient is again measured or the blood-flow probe reapplied, in order to verify or check the improvement.

Although *blind endarterectomy* has been used successfully on many occasions in the past (see Table 6.2), this technique is subject to many inaccuracies, and is not recommended.[70] It is essential to the performance of any endarterectomy that the normal arterial lumen distal to the reconstructed segment should be fully opened and carefully checked for raised flaps, detached areas of intima or accretions of thrombus. Given the limited exposure and short lengths of available vessel in this type of operation, these principles cannot be observed where reconstruction of the visceral arteries is concerned.

The indirect approach

By this is meant procedures designed to revascularize the intestine which do not encroach on the origin of the coeliac axis or SMA. These have the great advantages of avoiding the need to open the chest, and at the same time of steering clear of the difficult anatomical territory around the origin of the great vessels.

The standard incision is a long left paramedian, extending from just to the left of the xiphisternum to a point half-way between the umbilicus and the symphysis pubis. The peritoneum is opened and the abdominal contents carefully explored in the standard order.

Assuming that no other lesion has been found and that all is well within the peritoneal cavity, the revascularization is proceeded with, according to the site of the main lesion.

Occlusion of the coeliac axis.   This is dealt with by utilizing the splenic artery which, following removal of the spleen, is a convenient channel for retrograde irrigation of the coeliac territory. The artery may be implanted into the aorta, or a bypass may be inserted between it and the aorta or common iliac artery. In either case, the object is achieved of perfusing the coeliac axis distal to the occlusion or stenosis from an area of higher pressure.

A more usual situation is *a stenosis or occlusion of the SMA*. In fact, if normal arterial pressure is restored to the SMA territory, a coexistent lesion of the coeliac axis can be ignored, as the collaterals will have been developed to such an extent that adequate perfusion of the upper zone is assured.

There are various methods of revascularization of the SMA, both of which require the same exposure (see Fig. 6.11). To achieve this, the transverse colon is lifted upwards out of the wound and its mesentery incised over the origin of the middle colic artery. This vessel is then followed upwards to the main trunk of the SMA, which is then carefully freed from its companion vein. The SMA is mobilized up and down over some 3–4 cm, carefully preserving each intestinal artery as it is encountered, until a sufficient length has been mobilized for it to lie comfortably against the aorta (Fig. 5.9).

The peritoneum overlying the abdominal aorta is then incised and reflected medially and laterally, so as to expose the whole circumference of the vessel for 5 cm. If the aorta is of large calibre (4 cm or more in diameter) then it will usually be possible to effect the side-to-side anastomosis by application of a side-clamp to the aorta, allowing flow to proceed downwards (Fig. 6.9a). Usually, however, the diameter of the aorta is not big enough to allow the anastomosis to be performed comfortably in this way, and it is necessary to occlude it completely. This involves circumferential dissection of a 5-cm length of aorta, the lumbar branches being controlled with thread snares or bulldog clips (Fig. 6.9b).

It is wise, whenever the aorta is completely occluded, to protect the renal circulation by transfusing 20 g of mannitol intravenously.

Having controlled the aorta and SMA, the two vessels are approximated without tension by manipulating the controlling clamps, and a 2-cm longitudinal arteriotomy made in each of them. A stay-suture of 0000 synthetic cardiovascular material connects the arteriotomies at each end, and a continuous running suture completes the posterior layer (Fig. 6.10a). As the end of this layer is reached, the suture is tied and the anterior layer then

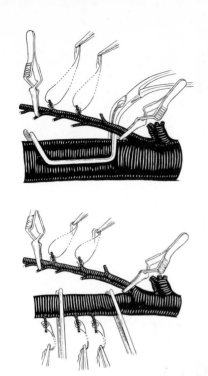

Fig. 6.9. Arterial reconstruction for chronic midgut ischaemia: clamping of aorta and control of branches of SMA: (a) with aorta of large calibre; (b) with aorta of small calibre.

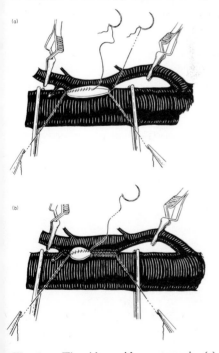

Fig. 6.10. The side-to-side anastomosis: (a) posterior suture line; (b) anterior suture line.

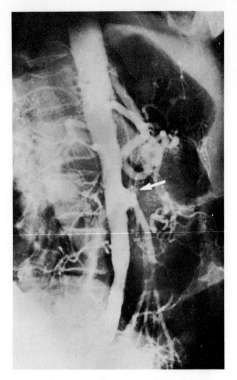

Fig. 6.11. Postoperative angiogram following side-to-side anastomosis between aorta and SMA. (The arrow demonstrates the site of the anastomosis.)

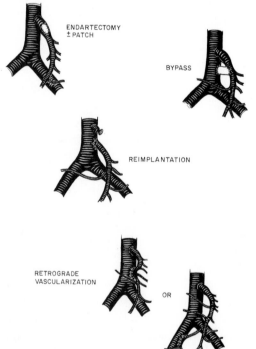

Fig. 6.12. Alternate techniques of visceral arterial reconstruction.

completed (Fig. 6.10b). Before final closure, clamps are briefly released from aorta and SMA in order to flush out any accumulated clot or debris. The anastomosis is then rapidly closed and the clamps removed, following which pressure measurements are again recorded.

An interesting finding during the performance of this type of anastomosis is that whereas the aorta is usually thickened and atheromatous, the part of the SMA used for the anastomosis, which lies distal to the block, is thin, supple and healthy. This illustrates the protective effect of a proximal arterial stenosis on the distal arterial tree, and helps to explain the relative rarity of atheromatous stenoses in the intestinal vessels themselves. There is some evidence to suggest that, in the lower limb, restoration of a normal distal pressure by means of an arterial reconstruction deprives the smaller vessels of this type of protection, so that they begin to develop plaques of atheroma. There is as yet no information forthcoming as to whether this process operates in the mesenteric circulation.

This operation (side-to-side aorto-SMA anastomosis) is safe and simple to carry out, and is of wide general applicability. The size of the stoma which can be obtained is illustrated in Fig. 6.11. Alternative methods of SMA reconstruction are illustrated in Fig. 6.12.

The coeliac axis compression syndrome

In 1963 Harjola[30] reported from Finland the case of a 57-year-old man who had complained for 10 years of colicky epigastric pains following meals, and who was found on clinical examination to have an arterial bruit in the upper abdomen. A lateral aortogram demonstrated stenosis of the origin of the coeliac axis. At operation it was found that the artery itself was normal, but that it was compressed by the fibres of the median arcuate ligament of the diaphragm. Division of these fibres abolished the palpable thrill and audible bruit and was followed by complete relief of the patient's pain when he was seen 2 months later.

Harjola was impressed by the similarity of this pain to 'classical' intestinal angina as described above, but was careful not to impute the symptoms to a reduction in blood supply, postulating rather a neural origin, due to fibrosis of the coeliac ganglion.

The concept of coeliac axis compression causing ischaemia of the upper abdominal viscera quickly caught on, however, and further cases were brought to light and operated upon. Thus Vollmar[87] and Gautier[29] each treated 2 patients by division of fibrous tissue, muscular bands and sympathetic nerves, with complete relief of symptoms. Dunbar et al.[22] then described a series of 21 patients, all of whom had epigastric pain after meals, associated with a systolic bruit. In 15 of these a lateral aortogram disclosed compression of the coeliac axis and this was confirmed in 13 at laparotomy. Although no very high pressure gradients were recorded across the stenoses, it was felt that there was impairment of flow, and indeed all these patients were relieved of their symptoms after division of the median arcuate ligament.

Table 6.2 The cœliac axis compression syndrome

Reference	No. of patients		Operations		Follow-up period (months)	Results
	Male	Female	Decompression	Reconstruction		
Harjola, 1963[30]	(2)		2		unstated	2 symptomless
Vollmar et al., 1964[87]	1	1			"	2 symptomless
Gautier et al., 1965[29]	2		2		"	unstated
Dunbar et al., 1965[22]	(27)		13 (+2)		unstated	2 unchanged
Drapanas & Bron, 1966[21]	(17)		1	1	unstated	2 symptomless
Snyder et al., 1967[80]		2	2		"	2 symptomless
Schmidt & Schimanski, 1967[76]	1	3				
Harjola & Lahtihaju, 1968[32]	3	13	11		6–50	9 symptomless / 3 improved / 1 unchanged
Marable et al., 1968[54]	3	27	25		12–48	18 symptomless / 4 improved / 3 unchanged
Lord et al., 1968[51]	3	9	4	8	"	11 symptomless / 1 unchanged
Fadhli, 1968[27]	1		1		8	1 symptomless
Deutsch, 1968[19]	1	2	1		unstated	1 symptomless
Carey et al., 1969[8]	1	1	2		"	2 symptomless

Reference						Outcome
Olivier et al., 1970[67]	5	1	6	2		6 symptomless (good)
Hivet et al., 1970[36]	(37)		unstated	,,	,,	
Jamieson & Greig, 1970[39]		1	1	,,	,,	1 symptomless
Cormier & Fontaine, 1970[12]	2	4	3	,,	,,	3 symptomless
Edwards et al., 1970[25]	2	5	unstated	,,	,,	2 symptomless / 3 unchanged
Curl et al., 1971[14]		1		1	15	1 symptomless
Mulder et al., 1971[66]	3	2	5		unstated	5 improved
Stanley & Fry, 1971[82]	5	10	12	1	,,	7 symptomless / 2 unchanged / 2 worse
Heberer et al., 1972[34]						
Evans, 1974[26]	10	40	47		6	39 symptomless / 8 unchanged
Beger et al., 1975[3]	4	4	6	1	6–50	4 symptomless
Kieny, 1976[45]	(30)		unstated		12–48	20 symptomless / 6 improved / 4 unchanged
TOTALS	47 (=286)	(113) 126	144 (+2)	14		131 symptomless / 18 improved / 26 unchanged or worse

Following this work, there have been a large number of cases reported in the literature, in which the coeliac axis (and, more rarely, the SMA) has been 'freed up', with relief of pain. Some authors have gone further than this and have actually carried out a reconstruction of the origin of the coeliac axis,* if simple division of the ligament did not appear to bring about an adequate improvement in pressure and flow. This case material is summarized in Table 6.2.

In an attempt to validate the concept of coeliac axis compression leading to ischaemia, there have been a number of laboratory studies. Thus Anderson et al.[1] studied the effect of graded occlusion of the coeliac axis with a Goldblatt clamp in a number of dogs, and demonstrated that as the lumen was progressively reduced, ulceration of the stomach and duodenum, and later actual infarction of the small bowel, occurred with increasing frequency. The number of survivors correspondingly declined, so that with a 75 per cent occlusion one-third of the animals had died at 2 days, and of 5 dogs undergoing a total occlusion, none survived. Stanley and Fry[81] studied the effect of chronic coeliac axis occlusion on *d*-xylose absorption, following the challenge of a meat meal. It is already known that no change in xylose absorption occurs under standard conditions following complete chronic occlusion of the SMA[55] but the authors felt that in the postabsorptive state the situation might be different, and indeed were able to demonstrate some impaired absorption in the 7 dogs they studied.

The challenge

While there remains a substantial body of surgical opinion which is convinced that the coeliac axis compression syndrome is a genuine entity, which can be completely relieved by division of the median arcuate ligament, others do not share this view. The earliest note of caution was struck by Reuter and Olin,[72] reporting from Lund, who examined 720 aortograms carried out between 1959 and 1965 in their department: 17 cases of coeliac axis stenosis or occlusion were picked out, of whom 5 had no abdominal symptoms and 7 had other types of pathology to account for their abdominal pain. Of the remaining 5 patients, 2 had cirrhosis and 1 was thought to have a peptic ulcer. The remaining 2 demonstrated stenosis of the inferior mesenteric artery as well as the coeliac axis, and, largely by exclusion, are presumed to be genuine cases of visceral ischaemia.

The following year, Drapanas and Bron[21] reported their 17 patients with coeliac axis stenosis or occlusion, of whom 6 were asymptomatic and 6 were suffering from gross intra-abdominal surgical pathology. Of the remaining 5, 1 patient underwent splenoaortic anastomosis, with no effect on the symptoms; in another, the coeliac axis was freed up by division of adhesions, but again the symptoms continued unabated. The remaining 3 patients all had extensive psychiatric problems.

This work was followed up by Bron and Redman,[7] who found a 17 per cent incidence of stenosis of the coeliac and mesenteric vessels in 713 aortograms, although none of their patients had symptoms resembling intestinal

* See References 6, 7, 8, 12, 14, 19, 21, 24, 25, 26, 27, 33, 36, 39, 46, 51, 54, 65, 66, 72, 75, 80, 82, 85.

angina. Interestingly, a rather larger proportion (49 per cent) of those patients with an isolated coeliac axis stenosis had symptoms than did those with multiple lesions. Edwards *et al.*[25] found that, of 200 healthy medical students, 13 had epigastric bruits of whom 1 complained of dyspepsia, whereas of 25 dyspeptics 1 had a bruit; 7 patients who had pain, bruit and a positive angiogram were offered operation, of whom 2 refused. Of the 5 patients operated upon, 2 lost their symptoms but the remainder were unchanged or worse. These authors were the first to measure pressure and flow during the operation, and were unable to correlate these with either preoperative symptoms or postoperative result. The frequency of asymptomatic stenosis of the coeliac axis has been further confirmed by Cornell[13] and Colapinto.[11]

A powerful onslaught on the whole idea of coeliac axis compression was mounted by Szilagyi,[86] who, following an extensive review of the literature, pointed out the variable nature of the symptoms described, the uncertainty of its relationship to 'true' intestinal angina resulting from SMA occlusion, and the lack of objective measurements recorded in the literature. These authors emphasized the fact that the postulated fault in coeliac axis compression was ischaemia, and consequent dysfunction, of the small bowel. No one had seriously suggested that there was any disturbance in function in the stomach, as this organ has an abundantly rich collateral blood supply, and it is within the experience of every general surgeon that it can be extensively devascularized without any impairment of function.[2] The theory is that the collateral vessels which develop as a result of coeliac artery stenosis 'steal' blood from the midgut loop, thus causing intestinal angina. However, the symptoms reported in the literature are of extreme variability, even if they are adequately described, which is by no means always the case. The only constant symptom is abdominal pain, but this is of quite unpredictable character, duration and relationship to meals. The so-called 'typical' pain is in fact only reported in 40 per cent of the total number of patients. Similarly, weight loss and diarrhoea are rare findings, and malabsorption, when looked for, is almost never present. The results of pressure and flow studies are equally equivocal. It is noteworthy that among the patients described there is a high incidence of psychological problems and of multiple previous abdominal explorations. Furthermore, a number of patients had additional rather more mundane abdominal problems such as peptic ulcer and gall-bladder disease, which might well have contributed to or even been entirely responsible for the symptoms, and certainly treatment of these conditions is as plausible a reason for the disappearance of pain as is the (possibly irrelevant) division of the median arcuate ligament.

Szilagyi and his associates go on to analyse their own clinical material. Examination of 200,000 new hospital admissions from 1965 to 1971 failed to reveal any case of supposed coeliac artery compression syndrome which satisfied them as showing a combination of angina, radiologically demonstrated coeliac artery stenosis and weight loss, and which was reversed by division of the median arcuate ligament. They did, however, find 24 cases in which coeliac axis compression had been considered as causing pain, other abdominal pathology having been ruled out. Additionally, on reviewing 157 unselected abdominal angiograms they found a 49 per cent incidence of coeliac axis stenosis. Interestingly, the incidence of stenosis was more or less evenly distributed over patients with and without abdominal pain and with and without gastrointestinal disease.

More recently Evans[26] has carried out a long-term evaluation of the 'coeliac band syndrome', studying 71 patients aged from 13 to 68 treated between the years 1963 and 1971. All of these patients had had a long history of abdominal pain and 70 per cent of them had undergone previous abdominal surgery. Of 59 patients traced from the original 71, 47 had undergone division of the median arcuate ligament (in 3 a cholecystectomy had been performed in addition), and 12 had been treated conservatively. At the initial follow-up examination which was carried out less than 6 months after the operation, 39 patients were free of symptoms and in 8 the situation was unchanged. However, at the later follow-up of 40 of these patients carried out at 3–11 years after the surgical procedure, the picture was very different. Of 18 patients who were asymptomatic, 13 had been reoperated upon for other abdominal conditions such as gall-bladder disease, peptic ulcer or subacute obstruction, leaving only 5 who ascribed their maintained improvement to the operation on the arcuate ligament. There were 4 patients who still had some symptoms though were somewhat improved, and 22 had in fact reverted to their original preoperative condition; 2 of these were subsequently rid of their pain by a cholecystectomy.

Of the 12 patients not subjected to surgery, 9 were asymptomatic, 1 was improved and 2 had retained their symptoms. It was interesting that there was no correlation between the condition of the patient at the original presentation and the achieved result at late follow-up.

Conclusions

It is clear from the statistics in Tables 6.1 and 6.2, as well as from a considerable amount of unpublished anecdotal material, that a number of patients with a combination of upper abdominal pain, epigastric bruit and narrowed origin of their visceral arteries do express gratitude following arterial reconstruction or division of the median arcuate ligament of the diaphragm. However, it is very difficult to go beyond this point and to prove that the pain is caused by diminished blood flow, that this interferes with function, and that the symptoms and the dysfunction are cured by surgery.

The placebo effect of a major operation, particularly when carried out by an attentive, enthusiastic and positive-minded surgeon, is enormous. It is fallacious to suppose that an operation is curative simply because the patient tells the surgeon that he feels better after it, and the history of surgery is littered with inappropriate procedures which have been evaluated in this way. Surgical success can only be evaluated on strict criteria.

1. *There must be a constant and definitive syndrome*, so that all can agree that they are treating the same problem. The 'atypical' case, therefore, cannot by definition exist. This certainly does not apply to chronic intestinal

ischaemia, in which the published series have included patients with widely differing modes of presentation and complaint.

2. *There must be a constant and definitive structural or functional abnormality*, which it is intended to correct. Extensive anatomical and radiological studies have shown that narrowing of the visceral arteries is a common finding in all manner of people with and without symptoms, and must therefore be considered as an anatomical variant rather than a pathological abnormality. Also, no consistent pattern of dysfunction has ever been demonstrated in the alimentary tract, resulting from such lesions. This applies both to haemodynamic studies and to measurements of absorption and excretion. In the few instances where such measurements have been made, these have failed to correlate either with the patients' symptoms or with the results of surgery.

3. *The abnormality must be abolished following the operation.* It is not enough to abolish the symptoms. What is necessary is to show a measurable disturbance of function which has been corrected. Such has yet to be found in chronic SMA occlusion, and this applies with even more force with regard to the coeliac artery compression syndrome.

Because of these fundamental objections, the tide of surgical opinion has now swung strongly against the concept that isolated narrowing of the origin of the coeliac axis is responsible for symptoms, or that operations designed to relieve it retain validity. To prove a negative is impossible, and indeed no one can say that division of the median arcuate ligament is in every case an irrelevant operation. However, in the author's view, the burden of proof that this major surgical intervention is beneficial rests with its proponents.

Atheromatous occlusion of the SMA, particularly in combination with other arterial stenoses, is in a different category, because there is much circumstantial evidence that such lesions can be dangerous. However, they are not always so, and as yet no test exists which will distinguish the clinically important from the clinically irrelevant mesenteric arterial block. Our own experience is summarized in Fig. 6.13.

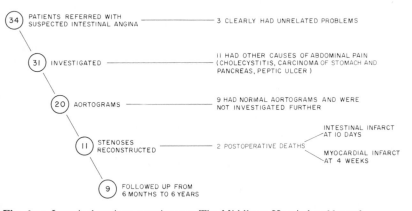

Fig. 6.13. Intestinal angina: experience at The Middlesex Hospital 1966–1976.

References

1   Anderson, M. C., Schiller, W. R., Suwa, M. and Geurking, R. E. (1968). Morphologic effects of graded celiac artery ischemia. *Bulletin de la Société Internationale de Chirurgie* **27**: 468–477.

2   Appleby, L. H. (1953). The celiac axis in the expansion of the operation for gastric carcinoma. *Cancer* **6**: 704–712.

3   Beger, H. G., Meves, M., Apitzsch, D., Kraas, E. and Bittner, R. (1975). Diagnose und operative Behandlung bei Arteria-Coeliaca-Kompression. *Deutsche Medizinische Wochenschrift* **100**: 464–471.

4   Bergan, J. J., Dry, L., Conn, J. and Trippel, O. H. (1969). Intestinal ischemic syndromes. *Annals of Surgery* **169**: 120–126.

5   Berman, L. G. and Russo, F. R. (1950). Abdominal angina. *New England Journal of Medicine* **242**: 611–613.

6   Bobbio, A. (1968). La syndrome del canale aortico del diaframma, stenosi da compressione del tronco celiaco. *Omnia Medica* **46**: 595–600.

7   Bron, K. M. and Redman, H. C. (1969). Splanchnic artery stenosis and occlusion. *Radiology* **92**: 323–328.

8   Carey, J. P., Stemmer, E. A. and Connolly, J. E. (1969). Median arcuate ligament syndrome. *Archives of Surgery* **99**: 441–446.

9   Carucci, J. J. (1953). Mesenteric vascular occlusion. *American Journal of Surgery* **85**: 47–51.

10 Chiene, J. (1869). Complete obliteration of the coeliac and mesenteric arteries: the viscera receiving their blood supply through the extrapyramidal system of vessels. *Journal of Anatomy and Physiology* **3**: 65–72.

11 Colapinto, R. F., McLoughlin, M. J. and Weisbrod, G. L. (1972). The routine lateral aortogram and the celiac compression syndrome. *Radiology* **103**: 557–661.

12 Cormier, J. M. and Fontaine, P. (1970). Sténose extrinsèque du tronc coeliaque. *Chirurgie* **96**: 453–456.

13 Cornell, S. H. (1971). Severe stenosis of the celiac axis. *Radiology* **99**: 311–315.

14 Curl, J. H., Thompson, W. N. and Stanley, J. L. (1971). Median arcuate ligament compression of the celiac and superior mesenteric arteries. *Annals of Surgery* **173**: 320.

15 Danis, J. and Frexinos, J. (1973). Aspects etiopathogéniques des sténoses non tumorales de l'intestin grêle. *Revue Médicale de Toulouse* **9**: 277–288.

16 Dardik, H., Soleidenberg, B., Parker, J. G. and Hurwitt, E. S. (1965). Intestinal angina with malabsorption treated by elective revascularization. *Journal of the American Medical Association* **194**: 1206–1210.

17 Delmont, J. P. (1965). L'insuffisance artérielle dans les territoires du tronc coeliaque et des mésenteriques supérieure et inférieure. *Journal de Chirurgie* **101**: 213–236.

18 Derrick, J. R., Pollard, H. S. and Moore, R. M. (1959). The pattern of arteriosclerotic narrowing of the celiac and superior mesenteric arteries. *Annals of Surgery* **149**: 684–690.

19 Deutsch, V. (1968). Compression of the coeliac trunk and the angiographic evaluation of its hemodynamic significance. *Clinical Radiology* **19**: 309–314.

20 Dick, A. P., Graff, R., Gregg, D., Peter, N. and Sarner, M. (1967). An arteriographic study of mesenteric arterial disease: large vessel changes. *Gut* **8**: 206–211.

21 Drapanas, T. and Bron, K. M. (1966). Stenosis of the celiac artery. *Annals of Surgery* **164**: 1085–1091.

22 Dunbar, J. D., Molnar, W., Beman, F. F. and Marable, S. A. (1965). Compres-

sion of the celiac trunk and abdominal angina. *American Journal of Roentgenology* **95**: 731–736.

23 Dunphy, J. E. (1936). Abdominal pain of vascular origin. *American Journal of Medical Science* **192**: 109–111.

24 Edwards, A. J. (1969). Coeliac axis compression syndrome. *Proceedings of the Royal Society of Medicine* **62**: 488–490.

25 Edwards, A. J., Hamilton, J. D., Nichol, W. D., Taylor, G. W. and Dawson, A. M. (1970). Experience with coeliac axis compression syndrome. *British Medical Journal* **1**: 342–345.

26 Evans, W. E. (1974). Long-term evaluation of the celiac band syndrome. *Surgery* **76**: 867–871.

27 Fadhli, H. A. (1968). Congenital diaphragmatic obstruction of the aorta and celiac artery. *Journal of Thoracic and Cardiovascular Surgery* **55**: 431–433.

28 Fry, W. J. and Kraft, R. O. (1963). Visceral angina. *Surgery, Gynecology and Obstetrics* **117**: 417–421.

29 Gautier, R., Barrié, J. and Sarrazin, R. (1965). Les angors abdominaux non athéromateux. *Lyon Chirurgical* **61**: 893–894.

30 Harjola, P. T. (1963). A rare obstruction of the coeliac artery—report of a case. *Annales Chirurgiae et Gynaecologiae Fenniae* **52**: 547–550.

31 Harjola, P. T. (1967). Coeliac axis constriction and abdominal angina. *Bulletin de la Société Internationale de Chirurgie* **27**: 464–467.

32 Harjola, P. T. and Lahtihaju, A. (1968). Celiac axis syndrome. *American Journal of Surgery* **115**: 864–869.

33 Heard, G., Jefferies, J. D. and Peters, D. K. (1963). Chronic intestinal ischaemia. *Lancet* **2**: 975–977.

34 Heberer, G., Dostal, G. and Hoffmann, K. (1972). Zur Erkennung und operativen Behandlung der Chronischen Mesenterialarterieninsuffizienz. *Deutsche Medizinische Wochenschrift* **97**: 750–754.

35 Herlinger, H. (1972). Angiography of the visceral arteries. *Clinics in Gastroenterology* **1**: 547–579.

36 Hivet, M., Legadec, B. and Poilleux, J. (1970). Les sténoses chroniques du tronc coéliaque. *Chirurgie* **96**: 483–486.

37 Imperati, L. and Tommaseo, T. (1960). *Chirurgia delle Arterie Mesenteriche*. Rome, Edizioni Mediche e Scientifiche.

38 Jackson, B. J. (1962). An approach to stenotic lesions of the S.M.A. *American Journal of Surgery* **104**: 86–91.

39 Jamieson, A. and Greig, J. H. (1970). Isolated celiac axis compression as a cause of visceral angina. *Canadian Medical Association Journal* **103**: 374–375.

40 Jaumin, P., Fastrez, J., Goenen, M., Raveau, A., Fiasse, R., Ponlot, R. and Dautrebande, J. (1974). Traitement chirurgicale de l'arterite mesenterique. *Acta Gastro-Enterologica Belgica* **37**: 413–428.

41 Johnson, C. C. and Baggenstoss, A. H. (1949). Mesenteric vascular occlusion. *Proceedings of the Staff Meeting of the Mayo Clinic* **24**: 649–656.

42 Julius, S. and Stewart, B. H. (1967). Diagnostic significance of abdominal murmurs. *New England Journal of Medicine* **276**: 1175–1178.

43 Keeley, F. X., Misanik, L. E. and Wirts, C. W. (1959). Abdominal angina syndrome. *Gastroenterology* **37**: 480–485.

44 Kieny, R., Cinqualbre, J., Pinke, R. and Jeanblanc, B. (1974). Chirurgie des lésions athéromateuses des artères digestives. In: *Chirurgie des Artériopathies Digestives*, pp. 141–148. Paris, Expansion Scientifique.

45 Kieny, R., Cinqualbre, J., Eisenmann, B. and Tongio, J. (1976). Ischémie mésentérique chronique. *Annales de Radiologie* **19**: 371–375.

46 Koikkalainen, K. (1971). Coeliac axis compression syndrome. *Annales Chirurgiae et Gynaecologiae Fenniae* **60**: 31–35.

47   Larson, R. E., Spittel, J. A. and Kirklin, J. W. (1963). Insufficiency of superior mesenteric artery. *Proceedings of the Staff Meeting of the Mayo Clinic* **38**: 436–440.

48   Lena, A., Tournigand, P. and Delmont, J. (1973). Treatment of chronic ischaemia of the small intestine. *Symposium (Nice) 1972*, pp. 80–91. Basel, Karger.

49   Lindner, H. H. and Kemprud, E. (1971). A clinico-anatomical study of the arcuate ligament of the diaphragm. *Archives of Surgery* **103**: 600–605.

50   Lipshutz, B. (1917). A composite study of the celiac axis artery. *Annals of Surgery* **65**: 159–169.

51   Lord, R. S. A., Stoney, R. J. and Wylie, E. J. (1968). Coeliac axis compression. *Lancet* **2**: 795–798.

52   Maljatzkaj, M. I. (1934). Uber die Atherosklerose der Baucharterien. *Beitrage für Pathologische Anatomie* **98**: 81–90.

53   Mandell, H. N. (1957). Abdominal angina—report of a case and review of the literature. *New England Journal of Medicine* **257**: 1035–1038.

54   Marable, S. A., Kaplan, M. F., Beman, F. M. and Molnar, W. (1968). Celiac axis compression syndrome. *American Journal of Surgery* **115**: 97–100.

55   Marston, A. (1964). Patterns of intestinal ischaemia. *Annals of the Royal College of Surgeons* **35**: 151–181.

56   Marston, A. (1972). Stenosis of the coeliac axis and superior mesenteric artery. *Annals of the Royal College of Surgeons* **50**: 327–328.

57   Marston, A., Kieny, R., Szilagyi, D. E. and Taylor, G. W. (1976). Intestinal ischemia. *Archives of Surgery* **111**: 107–112.

58   Masson, N. L. and Stayman, J. W. (1962). Intestinal angina. *American Journal of Surgery* **104**: 500–505.

59   Matthews, J. G. W. and Love, A. H. G. (1974). Interrelationship of mesenteric ischaemia and diarrhoea. *Proceedings of the Royal Society of Medicine* **67**: 12.

60   Mavor, G. E. and Lyall, A. D. (1962). Superior mesenteric artery stenosis treated by iliac-mesenteric arterial by-pass. *Lancet* **2**: 1143–1145.

61   Meyer, J. (1924). Intermittent claudication involving the intestinal tract. *Journal of the American Medical Association* **83**: 1414–1415.

62   Mikkelsen, W. P. (1957). Intestinal angina—its surgical significance. *American Journal of Surgery* **94**: 262–267.

63   Mikkelsen, W. P. and Zaro, J. A. (1959). Intestinal angina—report of a case with preoperative diagnosis and surgical relief. *New England Journal of Medicine* **260**: 912–914.

64   Mikkelsen, W. P. and Berne, C. J. (1962). Intestinal angina. *Surgical Clinics of North America* **42**: 1321–1328.

65   Morris, G. C., Crawford, E. S., Cooley, D. A. and De Bakey, M. E. (1962). Revascularization of the celiac and superior mesenteric arteries. *Archives of Surgery* **84**: 113–117.

66   Mulder, D. S., Rubush, J., Lawrence, M. S. and Ehrenheft, J. L. (1971). Celiac axis compression syndrome. *Canadian Journal of Surgery* **14**: 123–126.

67   Olivier, C., Rettori, R. and Dimaria, G. (1970). Stenoses non-atheromateuses et compressions du tronc celiaque. *Chirurgie* **96**: 471–481.

68   Passi, R. B. and Lansing, A. M. (1964). Experimental intestinal malabsorption produced by vascular insufficiency. *Canadian Journal of Surgery* **7**: 332–340.

69   Ranger, I. and Spence, M. P. (1962). Superior mesenteric artery occlusion treated by ileo-colic aortic anastomosis. *British Medical Journal* **2**: 95–97.

70   Reiner, L. (1964). Mesenteric arterial insufficiency and abdominal angina. *Archives of Internal Medicine* **114**: 765–772.

71   Reul, G. J., Wukash, D. C., Sandiford, F. M., Chiarillo, L., Hallman, G. L.

and Cooley, D. A. (1974). Surgical treatment of abdominal angina—report of 25 patients. *Surgery* **75**: 682–689.

72   Reuter, S. R. and Olin, T. (1965). Stenosis of the celiac artery. *Radiology* **85**: 617–627.

73   Reuter, S. R. (1971). Accentuation of celiac compression by the median arcuate ligament of the diaphragm during deep expiration. *Radiology* **98**: 561–564.

74   Rob, C. G. (1966). Surgical disease of the celiac and mesenteric arteries. *Archives of Surgery* **93**: 21–32.

75   Rob, C. and Snyder, M. (1966). Chronic intestinal ischemia: a complication of surgery of the abdominal aorta. *Surgery* **60**: 1141–1145.

76   Schmidt, H. and Schimanski, K. (1967). Die Stenose der Arteria Coeliaca—ihre Diagnose und Klinische Bedeutung. *Fortschritte Röntgenstrahlen* **106**: 1–12.

77   Schnitzler, J. (1901). Zur Symptomatologie des Darmarterienverschlusses. *Münschen Medizinische Wochenschrift* **98**: 552.

78   Sedlacek, R. A. and Bean, W. B. (1957). Abdominal angina. The syndrome of intermittent ischaemia of mesenteric arteries. *Annals of Internal Medicine* **46**: 148–152.

79   Shaw, R. S. (1959). Vascular lesions of the gastrointestinal tract. *Surgical Clinics of North America* **39**: 1258–1262.

80   Snyder, M. A., Mahoney, E. B. and Rob, C. G. (1967). Symptomatic celiac artery stenosis due to constriction by the neurofibrous tissue of the celiac ganglion. *Surgery* **61**: 372–376.

81   Stanley, J. C. and Fry, W. R. (1970). Provocative impairment of dextrorotatory xylose absorption in chronic intestinal ischaemia. *Surgical Forum* **21**: 330–331.

82   Stanley, J. C. and Fry, W. J. (1971). Median arcuate ligament syndrome. *Archives of Surgery* **103**: 252–258.

83   Starzl, T. E. and Trippel, O. M. (1959). Reno-mesenteri-aorto-iliac thromboendarterectomy in patient with malignant hypertension. *Surgery* **46**: 556–564.

84   Stoney, R. J. and Wylie, E. J. (1966). Recognition and surgical management of visceral ischemic syndromes. *Annals of Surgery* **164**: 714–722.

85   Sutton, R. A. L. (1967). Coeliac axis stenosis. *Proceedings of the Royal Society of Medicine* **60**: 139–141.

86   Szilagyi, D. E., Rian, R. L., Elliott, J. P. and Smith, R. F. (1972). The celiac artery compression syndrome: does it exist? *Surgery* **72**: 849–863.

87   Vollmar, J., Hartnet, H., Hasse, M., Schröder, E. and Coerper, H. G. (1964). Das Chronische Verschluss-syndrom der Eingeweide—Schlagadern. *Langenbecks Archiv für Klinische Chirurgie* **305**: 473–490.

88   Watt, J. K., Watson, W. C. and Haase, S. (1967). Chronic intestinal ischaemia. *British Medical Journal* **2**: 199–201.

89   Webb, W. R. and Hardy, J. D. (1962). Relief of abdominal angina by vascular graft. *Annals of Internal Medicine* **57**: 289–294.

90   Zahn, D. G. H. and Goerttler, K. (1971). Uber die Sklerose der Eingeweide Arterien. *Archiv für Kreislaufforschung* **64**: 235–271.

91   van Zyl, J. J. W. and du Toit, F. D. (1966). Superior mesenteric artery occlusion treated by common iliac-ileocolic anastomosis. *British Journal of Surgery* **53**: 522–524.

7

Focal Ischaemia of the Small Intestine: Ischaemic Stricture

Introduction

The fact that insufficiency of arterial supply can produce first inflammation and, later, ulceration and stenosis of a loop of small intestine has been known since the eighteenth century.[16, 48] It was confirmed in the laboratory in 1909 by Bolognesi,[7] who demonstrated that interference with small vessels led to oedema of the intestinal wall and infiltration of small round cells into the submucosa, later followed by the formation of a fibrous stricture. During this century there has been a great increase in the incidence both of inflammatory bowel disease and of degenerative conditions of the vascular system, and interest has begun to focus on ischaemia as a pathological process which can evoke a spectrum of responses in the small bowel, which may mimic Crohn's disease and other similar conditions.

The whole subject was carefully reviewed by Raf,[45] who examined the records of 12 surgical services in the Stockholm area over the period 1954–1965. He was able to trace 9,536 patients with non-malignant small bowel disease, of whom 95 (1 per cent) had presented with a non-inflammatory stricture. Of these patients, 59 had cardiovascular problems and had been under treatment for arterial hypertension and 14 had received radiotherapy to the pelvis, while the remainder had histories of strangulated hernia, abdominal trauma, internal haemorrhage or mesenteric vascular occlusion. In 1 case no cause could be found, and it is worthwhile noting that Williams[53] had drawn attention to the fact that non-occlusive ischaemia can give rise to intestinal stricture formation.

Causation

The following have been described in the literature as important causes of focal ischaemia of the small intestine:

1. Strangulation by external hernia or fibrous bands.[2, 9, 22, 34, 40, 50]
2. Trauma to the abdominal wall.[5, 10, 30, 37]
3. Acute ischaemia due to occlusion of the SMA, embolization to the small vessels or 'non-occlusive' mechanisms (see Chapter 4).[24, 38, 46, 53]
4. Inflammatory disease of the vessels of the gut wall.[15, 29]
5. Radiation injury.[1, 18, 27, 43, 52]
6. Action of enteric-coated potassium or other drugs on the mucosal circulation.[3, 6, 31, 32, 35, 47]

1. Strictures resulting from strangulation

The first description is probably that of Garengoet[16] who described some narrowing of the bowel associated with hernias, which he attributed to pressure from an ill-fitting truss. The condition was successfully operated upon by Vincent.[48] However, credit for the first definitive description of ischaemic damage following a strangulated hernia undoubtedly belongs to Guignard,[23] who described thickenings, constricting rings and loss of mucosa, encountered at the time of the operation for strangulated hernia. In 1892 Garré[17] produced his classic paper which contains the first description of delayed intestinal obstruction. The patient was a 27-year-old man who, 6 weeks after an operation for strangulated hernia at which compromised, though viable, gut had been returned to the abdomen, developed symptoms of intestinal obstruction, and at a second operation was found to have a 20-cm long stenosis which was densely adherent to other loops of small bowel. The condition is still sometimes referred to as 'intestinal stenosis of Garré', and has been reported on many occasions since.[5, 9, 12, 22, 34, 40, 50] Its frequency has undoubtedly decreased over recent years, partly due to the fact that inguinal hernias are now almost invariably treated at an early stage, before strangulation occurs, and also no doubt because attempted manual reduction of an obstructed hernia has become a discredited surgical manoeuvre.

None the less, Cherney[9] discovered 82 authenticated cases in the literature of stenosis following surgery for strangulation, and Vowles[50] and Cunningham and Regan[11] have reported further cases. As already mentioned, Raf found 8 examples in his Swedish series, of which 4 were the result of reduction of non-viable bowel from a hernial sac, and 4 resulted from strangulation by fibrous bands.

There is usually an interval of weeks or months between the vascular insult to the bowel and the development of symptomatic stricture.

2 Intestinal stricture following trauma

Blunt trauma to the abdominal wall may cause a haematoma to accumulate in the mesentery, or may actually separate mesentery from bowel over a variable length. In either case the result is severe local ischaemia. If a sufficient length of bowel is devascularized it will become necrotic, and perforate, leading to gross peritonitis. This may occur several days after an accident which initially appeared quite trivial. For this reason, among others, every patient with a closed injury to the abdomen must be regarded with suspicion, and minor complaints must be taken seriously and investigated with care, in order to exclude the presence of a loop of infarcted bowel.

Less complete degrees of ischaemia may be followed by the development of a fibrous stricture, which may not become manifest until months or even years after the original accident, although the usual interval between trauma and the development of obstruction is 2–12 weeks.[54] Such cases appear to be very rare. Although Gillet[19] was able to collect 48 from the world literature, in Raf's series from Stockholm there was only 1 traumatic stenosis in 95 cases.

3. Haemodynamic causes

Because of the very efficient collateral circulation of the small bowel (see Chapter 1), it is practically unknown for spontaneous occlusion of small vessels to lead to gangrene. Focal gangrene, when it occurs, is usually the result of SMA occlusion. This is in contrast to what has been described above in relation to trauma, where a tear or a haematoma in the mesentery destroys the collateral network. However, ischaemic ulceration, stenosis and stricture are not uncommon, and are quite often found at autopsy in patients who have suffered no alimentary symptoms during life. Additionally, a number of cases of acute small bowel obstruction are due to localized strictures, which histologically have all the characteristics of an infarction.[1, 8, 42, 49]

Again, a known vascular accident may later be followed by intestinal obstruction. In the cases reported by Rosenman and Gropper,[46] Pope and O'Neal[44] and Hawkins,[24] a mesenteric embolus had been treated conservatively and, presumably due to the development of an adequate collateral circulation, did not result in the death of the patient. After an interval of up to 10 weeks during which symptoms of the original abdominal crisis had passed off and the patient had recuperated, subacute small bowel obstruction developed as the fibrous tissue within the bowel wall began to organize and contract.

Apart from obstruction to the major arterial trunks, it is clear that focal ischaemic damage can occur from minor atheromatous emboli reaching the small intestinal vessels. This situation has been produced in the laboratory by the use of microspheres[6] and by cholesterol suspensions,[36] and there is some evidence that it can take place spontaneously in the human being. The occurrence of atheromatous emboli has been recognized ever since the classic description by Panum[41] of a ruptured plaque in the coronary artery of the sculptor Thorvaldsen, which had embolized into the myocardium, and caused his sudden death in a Copenhagen theatre. Gore[20] was the first to draw attention to the same process occurring in the gastrointestinal tract, and there have been several recorded cases since. Perhaps the best documented is that of Mulliken and Bartlett,[38] who resected a 17-cm length of fibrous and obstructed ileum from a 68-year-old woman, and demonstrated that the submucosal arteries were packed with the typical biconvex clefts left by cholesterol emboli.

Both the gross and microscopic appearances of focal ischaemia of the bowel may closely resemble Crohn's disease. This was emphasized by Hawkins,[24] who described a stenosis of the proximal jejunum occurring in a 74-year-old man 3 months after a myocardial infarction which had been complicated by a mesenteric embolus. At subsequent laparotomy the appearance of the bowel was identical with that of Crohn's disease though unfortunately the general condition of the patient did not allow of resection or biopsy, so that no histological information is available. However, in a case reported by Dingendorf[14] there was a double embolus into the distal branches of the SMA (demonstrated angiographically), and operation showed congestion and absent pulsation over a 70-cm length of small intestine. No resection was carried out at that time but 3 months later, following the development of severe obstructive symptoms, a grossly abnormal 40-cm length of ileum was removed. Careful histological examination showed the typical picture of Crohn's disease, with focal granulomata and epithelioid cells. The case is important and, as far as I know, unique. No one would suggest that the causation of Crohn's disease is a matter of impaired arterial supply, but it serves to draw attention to the fact that the histological behaviour of the bowel is not very versatile, and that the granulomatous response may perhaps be non-specific, and may occur in the face of widely differing types of challenge, including that of ischaemia.

Most varieties of intestinal ischaemia are found in adults, but an interesting series of small bowel infarcts occurring in Thai children was described by Headington *et al.*[25] In their 5 patients (2 of whom died), whose ages varied from 4 to 7, there was acute focal gangrene of the small intestine, with no associated arterial occlusion and no vasculitis. The authors were careful to exclude specific infection and, in particular, the presence of β-toxin-producing strains of *Clostridium perfringens*, as are seen in 'pig-bel' (see Chapter 5). The striking feature was the association of gross enlargement of the mesenteric lymph nodes in every case. The authors were unable to explain their findings.

4. Vasculitis

Many types of vascular disease, some of them extremely rare, can affect the gastrointestinal tract. The subject has been well covered by Feller[15] and by Kumar and Dawson,[29] and the reader is referred to their reviews. The more important conditions in this category are as follows.

Inflammatory conditions
Infective angiitis:
   typhoid
   tuberculosis
   syphilis
   leprosy
Specific arteritis of Crohn's disease
Buerger's disease (thromboangiitis obliterans)

Immune complex and collagen disorders
Systemic lupus erythematosus
Polyarteritis nodosa
Rheumatoid arthritis
Dermatomyositis
Sjogren's syndrome
Systemic sclerosis
Wegener's granuloma

Miscellaneous
Amyloidosis
Pseudoxanthoma elasticum
Ehlers–Danlos syndrome

Degos' disease (malignant papillitis)
Cogan's syndrome (non-syphilitic interstitial keratitis)

In most of these conditions, the bowel lesion is either a terminal event or simply forms part of a widespread symptom complex involving many organs and systems.

5. Radiation enteritis

Fibrous stricture of the intestine secondary to radiotherapy for carcinoma of the cervix was originally referred to by Jones in 1935,[27] and many thousands of cases have been reported since. The frequency of the complication varies from 1 to 12 per cent of the patients treated, and is becoming less with more accurate dosimetry and improved radiation techniques. The complication may appear from months to years after radiation therapy, but severe disturbances are comparatively rare.[28] In some 75–90 per cent of cases the large intestine and rectum are affected, following irradiation of uterine cancer. The most frequently affected zone of the bowel is some 8–14 cm from the anus. Due to its mobility, the small intestine is less commonly affected, and the usual site of damage here is from 6 to 10 cm from the ileocaecal valve. Jacobs[26] has reported a lesion in the ileum developing 32 year after radiotherapy, but most cases appear very much earlier than this. Sometimes the damage occurs progressively over a long period, and it is not unknown for successive operations to be required for the repeated development of strictures in areas of bowel which previously have been noted to be normal.[33]

Four syndromes have been described, the features of which may overlap.[27]

(a) *Acute necrotizing enteritis* occurs during therapy and presents with acute diarrhoea which may occasionally result in dehydration and collapse. This is due to a direct effect of the radiation on the mucosa. Wiernik[52] has shown that the villi become progressively shorter following irradiation, until a completely flat mucosa is produced, resulting in malabsorption and exudative enteropathy. Recovery occurs by the formation of flattened ridges rather than the normal finger-like processes. The timing of the processes of destruction and recovery is very variable. (b) *Subacute segmental enteritis* comes on at the end of therapy and presents with nausea, vomiting, diarrhoea and abdominal pain. This may clear up completely, or may lead to (c) *chronic enteritis*, characterized by long-continued episodic diarrhoea. Finally, as mentioned already, (d) *focal intestinal stricture* may develop, which can lead to complete obstruction.

Microscopically, a spectrum of changes is seen beginning with an infiltration with inflammatory cells and proceeding eventually to necrosis of the specialized layers of the wall, even at times ending in perforation. The bowel in most cases becomes thick and fibrous, and vascular adhesions develop between it and neighbouring structures. Vascular damage is patchy and in general confined to the area of stenosis. Although vessels in all layers of the bowel wall and mesentery are affected, by no means all the vessels are abnormal. The vascular changes vary from epithelial proliferation to focal medial necrosis or complete thrombotic occlusion.[43] The characteristic change is the accumulation of large foam cells beneath the intima and on the intimal side of the internal elastic lamina. This appears to be a specific diagnostic feature.

6. Ischaemia induced by drugs

In 1964 Lindholmer *et al.*[32] were surprised to encounter, in the space of less than 1 month, 4 cases of annular stricture of the small intestine, leading to obstruction. In view of the known rarity of this condition, they suspected that this sudden increase might be drug-induced, and set about investigating such a possibility. They discovered that the Stockholm hospitals had treated 16 similar patients during this period, making a total of 20, and further investigation showed that 17 of these patients had been taking tablets containing chlorothiazide and potassium. Two months later, Baker *et al.*[3] published an identical observation from the USA. More reports followed[13, 22, 31, 39, 47] which stimulated the interest of the Federal Food and Drug Administration in the problem. In a survey of 488 hospitals throughout the world, a total of 395 patients with small bowel ulceration was found, of whom 196 had been taking enteric-coated potassium chloride tablets and/or a thiazide diuretic.

It was not known at this point whether it was the thiazide, the potassium or the enteric coat which was in fact responsible for the production of the lesion, and neither was it known how the damage occurred. Experimental work followed, on the part of Lawrason,[31] who showed that intestinal ulceration could be produced in monkeys with thiazide and potassium chloride, but not with diuretic alone, and that the effect was probably dose-related. Further studies[35, 47] confirmed the damaging effect of high concentrations of potassium chloride, and have shown that the effect is greatly enhanced if SMA flow is reduced by constriction of the arterial lumen. Of the many thousands of patients taking this sort of medication, only a small minority develop ulceration, and it appears very much as though for structural damage to occur there must be a combination of pre-existing ischaemia and a high local concentration of potassium.[54]

The work of Boley *et al.*[6] shed some light on the evolution of the process. It appears that the first effect of a strong solution of potassium chloride is to cause venous spasm followed by thrombosis, leading to oedema of the submucosa and capillary damage. The resulting ischaemia goes on to mucosal loss, bacterial invasion, deposition of fibrous tissue and stricture formation. On occasion, the lesion may actually perforate and present with peritonitis. The results of the animal studies were reproduced in humans by Myers,[39] who injected hypertonic and isotonic solutions of potassium and sodium chloride into the intestinal lumen during resection procedures for colonic cancer.

Although the use of enteric-coated potassium tablets was undoubtedly responsible for the rapid increase in small bowel ulceration and stricture noted in the mid-1960s, this cannot be the whole story. The incrimination of potassium aroused much interest in the question of ulceration and stricture formation in the small bowel, and many cases were reported which otherwise would not have been brought to light. Davies and Bright-more[13] quote 12 patients with strictures, 6 of whom had received no potassium but who had been medicated with phenobarbitone, reserpine, phenylbutazone and steroids. Other series of case reports[12, 21, 51] have suggested similar implications. Whether or not such medication is relevant is a matter of speculation, but from what has already been said (Chapter 2) the small bowel circulation is sensitive to a great number of pharmacological agents, and intestinal ischaemia must be watched for as a possible complication of any newly introduced drug.

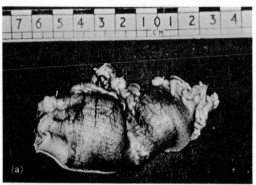

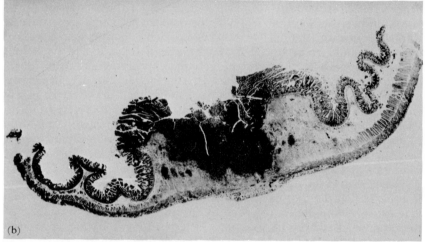

Fig. 7.1. Specimen of terminal ileum resected from a 57-year-old man who developed subacute small bowel obstruction while taking enteric-coated potassium tablets. (a) External aspect. (b) Transverse section (H & E × 25)

Clinical features of small intestinal strictures

Symptoms

The patient presents with the typical symptoms of subacute small intestinal obstruction; that is to say, colicky abdominal pain occurring usually some 2–3 hours after meals, and accompanied by nausea, occasional vomiting and distension. There may be episodes of diarrhoea. Fever, anorexia and gross loss of weight are unusual. Characteristically, the symptoms continue for a few weeks and months at a time, and then regress, to return at a later period with rather more intensity. Untreated, the condition progresses either to frank perforation of the bowel wall or to complete intestinal obstruction, in either case of which the patient will be admitted as a surgical emergency.

Naturally, a preceding history of strangulated hernia, ingestion of potassium tablets, episodes of ischaemia in other organs or radiation to the pelvis must be sought and carefully noted.

Physical examination

Physical examination of the abdomen is frequently quite normal, but may on occasion show a 'ladder pattern' of distension, with visible peristalsis and exaggerated bowel sounds. Except in very advanced cases, the serum biochemistry remains normal.

X-ray examination

X-ray examination will confirm the presence of dilated loops of jejunum with oedema of the wall and occasional fluid levels. A small bowel meal is perhaps the most useful investigation, as it will on occasion delineate the position of the stricture as well as confirming the diagnosis.

Management

Fluid losses are replaced, and anaemia corrected, before undertaking surgery for the obstructing lesion. The operation consists simply in resection of the stricture, with end-to-end anastomosis, and usually proceeds very simply along the standard lines. Naturally, if there is any question of a pre-existing lesion in the SMA, particular care must be taken to check the vascularity of the ends of the bowel. This will apply most strongly in postirradiation cases, where tissue healing may be seriously impaired. For this reason surgeons are reluctant to interfere with radiation strictures, but the fact must be faced that symptomatic intestinal obstruction can only be dealt with surgically, and provided that the anastomosis is constructed well back in healthy bowel, the operation should be reasonably safe. None the less, these wounds should never be closed without ample drainage in case a leak should occur.

References

1   Aune, E. F. and White, B. V. (1957). Gastrointestinal complications of irradiation for carcinoma of uterine cervix. *Journal of the American Medical Association* **147**: 831–834.

2   Avery, J. (1853). Almost complete obstruction of the small intestine from injury. *Transactions of the Pathological Society* **4**: 156–157.

3   Baker, D. R., Schrader, W. H. and Hitchcock, C. R. (1964). Small bowel ulceration apparently associated with thiazide and potassium therapy. *Journal of the American Medical Association* **190**: 586–590.

4   Barlow, D. (1961). Pathological changes in a jejunal graft used for oesophageal reconstruction. *Proceedings of the Royal Society of Medicine* **54**: 161–162.

5   Beringuier, M. (1877). Retrecissement fibreux de l'intestin grêle. *Bulletin de la Société Anatomique de Paris* **2**: 86–88.

6   Boley, S. J., Schults, L., Krieger, H., Schwartz, S., Elguezabal, A. and Allen, A. C. (1965). Experimental evaluation of thiazides and potassium as a cause of small bowel ulcer. *Journal of the American Medical Association* **192**: 763–768.

7   Bolognesi, G. (1909). De l'occlusion expérimentale des vaisseaux mésenteriques. *Zentralblatt für Chirurgie* **36**: 1641–1647.

8   Brookes, V. S., Windsor, C. W. O. and Howell, J. S. (1966). Ischaemic ulceration with stricture formation in the small bowel. *British Journal of Surgery* **53**: 583–585.

9   Cherney, L. S. (1958). Intestinal stenosis following strangulated hernia—review of the literature and report of a case. *Annals of Surgery* **148**: 991–993.

10   Courriades, H. (1949). Deux cas de sténose traumatique de l'intestin. *Mémoires de l'Académie de Chirurgie* **75**: 266–267.

11   Cunningham, W. L. and Regan, J. F. (1965). Fibrous stenosis of the small bowel and the role of ischemia. *Surgery* **58**: 488–496.

12   Danis, J. and Frexinos, J. (1973). Aspects etiopathogéniques des sténoses non-tumorales de l'intestin grêle. *Revue Médicale de Toulouse* **9**: 277–288.

13   Davies, D. R. and Brightmore, T. (1970). Idiopathic and drug-induced ulceration of the small intestine. *British Journal of Surgery* **57**: 134–139.

14   Dingendorf, W., Swart, B. and Haberich, H. (1971). Inkomplette Mesenterial gefässverschlüsse als mögliche Ursache der Enteritis regionalis Crohn. *Der Radiologe* **2**: 37–42.

15   Feller, E., Rickert, R. and Spiro, H. M. (1971). Small vessel disease of the gut. In: *Vascular Disorders of the Intestine*, pp. 483–509. Ed. by S. J. Boley. New York and London, Appleton-Century-Crofts.

16   Garengoet, R. J. C. de (1748). *Traité des Opérations de Chirurgie*, 3rd edn., Vol. 1, Huart. Paris, p. 286.

17   Garré, C. (1892). Ueber eine eigenartige Form von narbiger Darmstenose nach Brucheinklemmung. *Beiträge zur Klinischen Chirurgie* **9**: 187–197.

18   Gilles, M. and Skyring, A. (1967). Gastrointestinal complications of radiotherapy. *Australasian Radiology* **11**: 254–260.

19   Gillet, M., Phillipe, E. and Adloff, M. (1967). Les sténoses cicatricielles de l'intestin grêle après contusion de l'abdomen. *Journal de Chirurgie* **93**: 469–477.

20   Gore, I. and Collins, D. P. (1960). Spontaneous atheromatous embolization. *American Journal of Clinical Pathology* **33**: 416–418.

21   Greenblatt, M. and Goodman, H. (1959). Segmental jejunal stenosis of ischemic origin. *New England Journal of Medicine* **261**: 754–756.

22   Griswell, T. L. (1949). Complications of treatment of incarcerated hernia with vasodilatant drug. *Journal of the Indiana State Medical Association* **42**: 522–524.

23   Guignard, P. E. (1846). De Rétrécissement et de l'Oblitération de l'Intestin. *Thesis*, Paris University.

24   Hawkins, C. F. (1957). Jejunal stenosis following mesenteric artery occlusion. *Lancet* **2**: 121.

25 Headington, J. T., Sathornsumathi, S., Simark, S. and Sujatakond, W. (1967). Segmental infarcts of the small intestine and mesenteric adenitis in Thai children. *Lancet*, **1**: 802–806.

26 Jacobs, L. G. (1963). Unusual case of late irradiation damage to the ileum. *Radiology* **80**: 57–60.

27 Jones, T. F. (1935). Intestinal complications resulting from prolonged radium and x-ray irradiation for malignant conditions of pelvic organs. *American Journal of Obstetrics and Gynecology* **29**: 309–316.

28 Kott, I., Urca, I. and Kesler, H. (1971). Gastrointestinal complications after therapeutic irradiation. *Diseases of the Colon and Rectum* **14**: 200–215.

29 Kumar, P. J. and Dawson, A. M. (1972). Vasculitis of the alimentary tract. *Clinics in Gastroenterology* **1**: 719–745.

30 Küttner, H. (1930). Die Spätsschädigungen des Darmes nach stumpfer Bauchverlätzung. *Ergebnisse der Chirurgie und Orthopädie* **23**: 205–237.

31 Lawrason, F. D., Alpert, E., Mohr, F. L. and McMahon, F. G. (1965). Ulcerative obstructive lesions of the small intestine. *Journal of the American Medical Association* **191**: 641–645.

32 Lindholmer, B., Nyman, E. and Raf, L. (1964). Non-specific stenosing ulceration of the small bowel. *Acta Chirurgica Scandinavica* **128**: 310–311.

33 Localio, S. A., Stone, A. and Freidman, M. (1969). Surgical aspects of radiation enteritis. *Surgery, Gynecology and Obstetrics* **129**: 1163–1172.

34 Maass, V. (1895). Über die Entstahung von Darmen stenose nach Brucheinklemmerug. *Deutsche Medizinische Wochenschrift* **21**: 365–367.

35 Mansfield, J. B., Schoenfeld, F. B., Suwa, M., Geurkink, R. E. and Anderson, M. C. (1967). The role of vascular insufficiency in drug induced small bowel ulceration. *American Journal of Surgery* **113**: 608–614.

36 Marston, A., McCombs, L. and Lundqvist, E. (1962). Unpublished observations.

37 Moell, P. O. (1958). Posttraumatisk Colonstriktur. *Nordisk Medicin* **60**: 1834–1835.

38 Mulliken, J. B. and Bartlett, M. K. (1971). Small bowel obstruction secondary to atheromatous embolization. *Annals of Surgery* **174**: 145–150.

39 Myers, R. N., Brown, C. E. and Deaver, J. M. (1967). In vivo effect of potassium on small bowel. *Annals of Surgery* **166**: 693–703.

40 Obre, H. (1851). Disease of the intestine following strangulation eleven months previously. *Transactions of the pathological society* **3**: 96–97.

41 Panum, P. L. (1862). Experimentalle Beiträge zur Lehre von der Embolie. *Archiv für Pathologische Anatomie* **25**: 308–312.

42 Parenski, R. (1876). Intestinal stricture due to cicatrizing infarct. *Wiener Medizinische Jahrbuch* **275**.

43 Perkins, D. E. and Spjut, H. J. (1962). Intestinal stenosis following radiation therapy. *American Journal of Radiology* **88**: 953–966.

44 Pope, C. H. and O'Neal, R. M. (1956). Incomplete infarction of ileum simulating regional enteritis. *Journal of the American Medical Association* **161**: 963–964.

45 Raf, L. E. (1969). Ischaemic stenosis of the small intestine. *Acta Chirurgica Scandinavica* **135**: 253–259.

46 Rosenman, L. D. and Gropper, A. N. (1955). Small intestine stenosis caused by infarction: an unusual sequel of mesenteric artery embolism. *Annals of Surgery* **141**: 254–262.

47 Stahlgren, L. H., Dapena, A. and Roy, R. L. (1965). Ulcerogenic properties of enteric coated compounds in dogs. *Surgical Forum* **16**: 367–370.

48 Vincent (1781). Observations sur l'operation de Ran'hor. *Journal de Medicale et Chirurgie et Pharmacologie* **56**: 151.

49   von Brücke, H. (1935). Über Ischaemische Darmstenose. *Archiv für Klinische Chirurgie* **182**: 95–106.
50   Vowles, K. D. J. (1959). Intestinal complications of strangulated hernia incidence of ischaemic strictures. *British Journal of Surgery* **47**: 189–192.
51   Wayte, D. M. and Helwig, E. B. (1968). Small bowel ulceration—iatrogenic or multifactorial origin? *American journal of clinical pathology* **49**: 26–39.
52   Wiernik, G. (1966). Changes in the villous pattern of the human jejunum associated with heavy radiation damage. *Gut* **7**: 149–153.
53   Williams, L. F., Anastasia, L. S., Hasiotis, C. A., Bosniak, M. A. and Byrne, J. J. (1967). Non-occlusive mesenteric infarction. *American Journal of Surgery* **114**: 376–381.
54   Windsor, C. W. O. (1972). Ischaemic strictures of the small bowel. *Clinics in Gastroenterology* **1**: 707–717.

8

Ischaemic Colitis

Introduction

As was made plain in Chapter 4, the result of deprivation of blood supply, depending on its extent and duration, to a loop of intestine can range from full-thickness necrosis (gangrene) to a transient invasion by bacteria and inflammatory cells, which heals completely. Falls in blood flow which are insufficient to kill the bowel wall may none the less result in permanent damage to the mucosal and muscle layers, which become replaced by scar tissue, resulting in the formation of a fibrous stricture. All these haemo-dynamic events produce results which are interpreted by pathologists as 'inflammation' and closely resemble the products of infection and of local tissue immunity, and the concept of ischaemic colitis grew from the con-vergence of dissimilar medical disciplines, namely those of the vascular surgeon and the gastroenterologist. As has so often happened in medical history, the realization of a shared problem resulted in a new avenue of investigation and discovery.

Causes of colonic ischaemia (see Fig. 8.1)

Surgical interruption of the blood supply

Although the damaging effects of interference with the intestinal arterial supply had been recognized for many years, credit (if this is the right term to use for a surgical mistake!) is usually given to Lauenstein[56] as being the first to describe gangrene of the colon following a vascular accident. His patient developed a slough of the transverse colon after ligation of the middle colic artery in the course of a gastrectomy. With the develop-ment of radical surgery for cancer of the colon, surgeons became interested in high ligation of the arterial trunks, so as to achieve wider clearance of the lymphatics, and the risks of devitalization of anastomoses and stomata became a major preoccupation. The first successful ligation of the inferior mesenteric artery was recorded by Treves in 1898,[102] and further reports followed by Kummel,[53] Hartmann,[39] and Pope and Judd,[90] who recom-mended that in excision of the rectum the artery should be divided below its first sigmoid branch. Later, 'high ligation' of the IMA (i.e. at its aortic origin) became standard practice, but a note of warning was sounded by Goligher[33] who described a 25 per cent incidence of devitalization of the terminal colon following this manœuvre, and others[2, 38] reported similar complications and disasters. It became apparent that a crucial factor in the preservation of the colonic blood supply was the marginal artery to

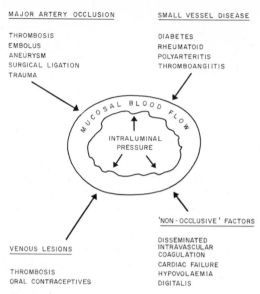

MAJOR ARTERY OCCLUSION

THROMBOSIS
EMBOLUS
ANEURYSM
SURGICAL LIGATION
TRAUMA

SMALL VESSEL DISEASE

DIABETES
RHEUMATOID
POLYARTERITIS
THROMBOANGIITIS

MUCOSAL BLOOD FLOW

INTRALUMINAL
PRESSURE

'NON-OCCLUSIVE' FACTORS

DISSEMINATED
INTRAVASCULAR
COAGULATION
CARDIAC FAILURE
HYPOVOLAEMIA
DIGITALIS

VENOUS LESIONS

THROMBOSIS
ORAL CONTRACEPTIVES

Fig. 8.1. Factors leading to ischaemia of the colon.

the colon, and that an arterial and lymphatic watershed existed at the splenic flexure where the middle and left colic arteries frequently fail to communicate[77] (see Chapter 2). A deficient marginal artery, an absent arteria anastomotica magna (Van Heller's artery) or unsuspected occlusive disease of the superior mesenteric artery may, either singly or in combination, imperil the blood supply of an anastomosis in the left colon.

From quite another area, surgeons interested in cardiovascular disease were beginning, in the early 1950s, to reconstruct the lower aorta, which frequently involved sacrifice of one or more of its visceral branches, in particular the inferior mesenteric artery. Cannon[13] reported a patient who died from unsuspected gangrene of the left colon 10 days following an emergency operation for aneurysm, and the first major report along these lines came from Smith and Szilagyi,[98] who described 12 cases of ischaemia of the descending colon in 120 aortic resections. Many cases have now been recorded and the incidence of colonic ischaemia following aortic surgery varies from 3 to 15 per cent, according to the care with which it is sought. The first cases to be reported were of frank gangrene, but subsequent study has shown that milder variants are common,[5, 34, 60, 73] Thus Bernstein and Bernstein[4] reported a patient who suffered a transient period of colonic inflammation following aneurysmectomy, and a similar case is illustrated in Fig. 8.8. Subsequent reports[6, 72, 79, 109, 110] have shown that aortic surgery can lead to the formation of a permanent fibrous stricture in the colon, without necrosis.

The IMA is often ligated as a necessary part of operations on the lower aorta and the large bowel, and obviously this is a perfectly safe manœuvre if the vessel is already occluded. Before a patent IMA is tied, however, the surgeon must satisfy himself as to the integrity of the marginal artery and of the SMA; if doubt exists, the vessel must be reimplanted into the

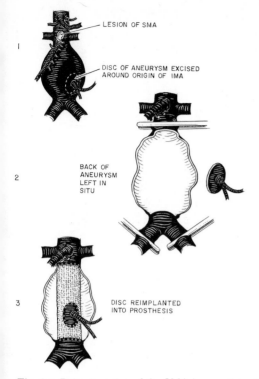

LESION OF SMA

DISC OF ANEURYSM EXCISED
AROUND ORIGIN OF IMA

1

BACK OF
ANEURYSM
LEFT IN
SITU

2

DISC REIMPLANTED
INTO PROSTHESIS

3

Fig. 8.2. Reimplantation of the SMA in resection of an aortic aneurysm.

aortic prosthesis[24, 95] (see Fig. 8.2). The whole question of colonic damage following aortic reconstruction has recently been reviewed by Johnson and Nabseth,[45] who found an over-all incidence of 99 cases in 6,100 patients at risk, or 1·6 per cent.

Radiological injury

The colon can also be damaged following free or selective abdominal angiography. This was first reported by Joyeux[46] and was well reviewed by Killen[50] who collected 15 cases from the literature, 3 of which exhibited inflammation only, the remaining 12 undergoing necrosis. Almost certainly the actual incidence at that time was higher as many milder cases would have passed unnoticed or unreported. It is not clear from this or other reports[82, 105] whether the contrast medium or the trauma of cannulation is to blame, or indeed whether the inferior mesenteric artery did not become blocked as a result of the angiography. Experimental work suggests that the gut is very tolerant of concentrated angiographic media, and the more recently introduced of these agents are probably much less toxic than those in use at the time of Killen's study

Table 8.1 Ischaemic colitis related to arterial occlusion

Reference	Sex and age of patient	Clinical presentation	Bowel lesion	Vascular lesion	Outcome
Gambee, 1937[29]	M/70	LIF pain and rectal bleeding	Ulceration left colon	Thrombosis of IMA	Resection. Death at 8 days
Huggard & Herstein, 1948[42]	F/20	LIF pain 24 hours postpartum	Infarction left colon	Thrombosis of IMA	Resection Recovery
Thompson, 1948[101]	M/55	Abdominal pain and diarrhoea	Gangrenous rectosigmoid	Intramural thrombosis of arteries and veins	Colostomy, exteriorization. Recovery
Cooling & Protheroe, 1958[19]	F/59	Abdominal pain, diarrhoea and blood	Mucosal congestion and ulceration of transverse colon	Thrombosis of middle colic artery	Resection. Recovery
McCourt, 1960[58]	M/51	LIF pain and bleeding	Infarction splenic flexure	Thrombosis of IMA	Resection. Death from gangrene of small bowel
Harrison & Croal, 1962[38]	M/70	LIF pain and bloody diarrhoea	Mucosal inflammation, later perforation and abscess	Occlusion of aorta and IMA	Death
Marston, 1962[64]	M/68	Abdominal pain, diarrhoea and blood	Congestion, fibrosis and ulceration of splenic flexure	Thrombosis of middle colic artery	Colostomy, resection. Recovery
Wald, 1964[103]	M/66	Pain and rectal bleeding	Gangrene of colon from hepatic flexure to pelvic floor	Aortic aneurysm with dissection of IMA	Two-stage proctocolectomy. Recovery
Payan et al., 1965[85]	F/70	Pain and bloody diarrhoea	Diagnosed as ulcerative colitis on	Occlusion of IMA	Death from cardiac failure

			showed ulcers, haemorrhagic inflammation		
Shippey & Acker, 1965[97]	F/67	Colic pains 5 years, recent acute episode with vomiting. Blood found in rectum	Thumb-printing around splenic flexure, later resolving to stricture	Narrowing of IMA, occlusion of left colic artery	Resection of stricture. Recovery
Dunbar, 1966[25]	M/45	Acute RIF pain 2 weeks following myocardial infarction	Thumb-printing in caecum	Embolus in ileocolic artery	Conservative treatment. Follow-up angiograms demonstrated collateral circulation. Recovery
Westcott, 1972[104]	F/63	Bleeding and diarrhoea	Thumb-printing around splenic flexure	Occlusion of left colic artery	Conservative treatment. Subsequent bariums became normal. Recovery
Lambana et al., 1973[54]	M/76	LIF pain and bloody diarrhoea	Stricture at splenic flexure, with tubular narrowing and sacculation	Atheromatous occlusion of sigmoid arteries	Resection of structure. Recovery.
Neto & Ribeiro, 1974[80]	M/78	LIF pain and vomiting	Mucosal inflammation on sigmoidoscopy. Gangrene of colon from splenic flexure to rectum	Occlusion of IMA	Resection. Recovery

Spontaneous Thrombosis of the colonic vessels

As already described (see Chapter 2), the inferior mesenteric artery is frequently narrowed or blocked at its origin by an atheromatous plaque,[15, 29, 32, 37] and this situation is usually well compensated by the development of collateral pathways. If the compensatory mechanisms fail, the colon is damaged and there are many recorded examples of this occurring as a result of acute occlusion of the artery, which are set out in Table 8.1. The changes described vary from gangrene (and, understandably, the earlier series are exclusively concerned with this) to the more recently familiar changes of 'thumb-printing', mucosal ulceration and stricture formation (see below). These features have all been produced in the experimental laboratory (see Chapter 4).

Small vessel disease

Often, the causative lesion is at subradiological level, in the intramural vessels. As in the small bowel, any condition which produces inflammation of minor arteries may result in mucosal damage. These include primary vascular disorders such as polyarteritis and Buerger's disease, systemic lupus erythematosus, rheumatoid arthritis and dermatomyositis.[61, 76] Also included in this group are Wegener's granuloma, anaphylactoid purpura and Degos' disease.[28] Perhaps one should also mention in this regard the effect of radiation on the colon, as may particularly occur following treatment of uterine carcinoma (see Chapter 7). Necrosis of the colon occasionally complicates renal transplantation,[86, 91] presumably as an indirect effect of immune suppression.

Atheromatous emboli from the aorta, and intimal thickening occurring in diabetes, have also been incriminated. It seems entirely logical that such conditions could lead to colonic ischaemia, but the written work in this area is largely speculative, and firm clinical reporting is hard to come by.

Low-flow states

The colon is subject to all the factors contributing to intestinal failure (see Chapter 5), and when its blood supply fails the resulting inflammatory damage will be more rapid and more metabolically harmful than a similar process in the small gut, due to the presence of pathogenic bacteria. Of particular importance in this connection are the Clostridia, which can be found in the colons of 1 in 3 healthy human subjects. As in the small bowel, predisposing factors include cardiac failure (particularly in association with digitalis intoxication, hypertension, diabetes and any condition which leads to disseminated intravascular coagulation (see Fig. 8.1)).

Obstruction

As already pointed out, blood flow in the wall of the intestine is dependent on intraluminal pressure, radial muscle tension and diameter, quite apart from vascular influences (see Fig. 8.1). The characteristic radiological and pathological changes of ischaemic colitis occur frequently in the segment of bowel immediately proximal to an obstructing carcinoma (the so-called 'stercoral' ulceration).[1, 41, 94] Sometimes, in fact, the clinical effects of the ischaemic lesion may be sufficiently severe as to mask the presence of the tumour.[7] Other factors leading to obstruction of the lumen of the large bowel, such as prolapse,[48] volvulus, adhesions or narrowing at the site of a colostomy,[100] may in the same way give rise to local ischaemic change.

Venous occlusion

Experimental studies[62] demonstrate that although interruption of the inferior mesenteric vein or one of its major tributaries produces very little effect, extensive venous thrombosis, as follows injections of thrombin, leads to a haemorrhagic type of infarction, with gross oedema. As this lesion matures, it comes to resemble even more closely the late results of arterial occlusion.

The clinician sees the lesion at a mature stage. By the time x-rays can be taken and histological material may be available, it may be impossible to decide whether the original causation of the infarct was on the arterial or the venous side. Circumstantial evidence to incriminate the oral contraceptive pill (which is known to have a selective influence on venous thrombosis elsewhere in the body) is not hard to come by,[21, 23, 52] though it must be admitted that no colon has ever been proven to have been damaged as a direct result of such medication. True the earlier reported series[65] of

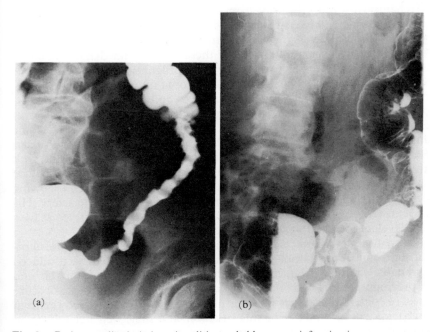

(a)   (b)

Fig. 8.3. Barium studies in ischaemic colitis: probable venous infarction in a young woman taking oral contraceptive: (a) on admission; (b) after 3 weeks.

patients with ischaemic colitis included no premenopausal females, whereas those reported since the introduction of oral contraceptives have included a limited number of young women, but this cannot be taken to be more than suggestive, and indeed the incidence of the condition in young men is becoming increasingly recognized,[17, 31, 80]

It would be surprising if venous disease of the colon were not in some measure responsible for mucosal pathology, but the association has yet to be proven (Fig. 8.3).

The concept of ischaemic colitis

The situation in the mid-1960s was that it was known that arterial injury brought about by a surgeon or a radiologist, spontaneous thrombosis of major or minor arteries, low-flow states, raised intraluminal pressure or blocked veins, could produce a spectrum of colonic disorders which varied from mild transitory inflammation to gangrene. The radiological and pathological changes invoked by ischaemia were established, and were beginning to be reproduced in the experimental laboratory.[8, 68] This prompted the suspicion that many unexplained cases of 'colitis' could perhaps be manifestations of arterial insufficiency.

For many years, gastroenterologists had been aware that their classification of acute inflammatory disease of the colon was insufficient to accommodate all observed cases. Specific infections, such as bacillary and amoebic dysentery or infestation by parasites, were readily understood. Mechanical disorders resulting from stricture or bands or muscle dysfunction as in the case of diverticular disease, formed another well defined category. The causation of the 'granulomata', namely ulcerative colitis and Crohn's disease, was not known but these were useful diagnostic labels in terms of natural history, pathology and prognosis. Many examples of acute colitis had been reported which did not fit into any established clinical category and in which the pathology was quite unlike Crohn's disease or ulcerative colitis. These had been given various names such as 'regional colitis',[11] 'acute segmental colitis'[49] and 'fibrous stenosis',[37] and some authors had in fact suggested a vascular basis for their cases, in particular Boley[8] who, in an important paper, described 5 patients presenting with abdominal pain and rectal bleeding, whose barium enemas showed 'thumb-printing' around the splenic flexure, exactly as is seen following deliberate or spontaneous occlusion of the inferior mesenteric artery. His patients recovered without specific treatment and were interpreted as having developed reversible vascular occlusions.

In 1966 we described[65] a series of 16 patients with an illness whose clinical, radiological and pathological features were identical to those produced by known vascular insufficiency in the colon. From a study of this and of previous material we concluded that a large number of hitherto obscure cases of colitis were in fact varieties of infarction. We developed the term 'ischaemic colitis' to describe this situation, and suggested a classification of the disease into gangrenous, stricturing and transient forms, according to the security of the ischaemia, at the same time laying down its clinical, radiological and pathological features. This concept became generally accepted, and many reports of cases of ischaemic colitis have appeared in the world literature during the subsequent decade.*

The clinical, radiological and pathological features are now well established and have been reproduced in the experimental laboratory by varying degrees of interruption of the arterial supply to the colon[68, 70] (see Chapter 3). However, to diagnose ischaemic colitis is to make a statement of quite a different order from a diagnosis of ulcerative colitis or Crohn's disease, because an underlying aetiology is implied. The difficulty is that angiograms by no means always demonstrate a vascular occlusion. This state of affairs is of course to be expected, in view of the known fact that approximately one-third of fatal intestinal infarcts occur in the absence of a defined vascular pathology (Chapter 5). None the less, when ischaemic colitis is diagnosed (as it often is) on the basis of a clinical story and a barium enema, without the opportunity of examining histological material, the clinician is open to the challenge that whatever has happened in the colon is not in fact the result of deficient blood flow. The situation is rather analogous to that of a myocardial infarct which is diagnosed on the evidence of the patient's symptoms, physical signs and electrocardiograph, but without a coronary angiogram.

Angiography in both these situations is not justified as a routine procedure, both because it is an invasive investigation which will not in itself influence treatment policy, and because a normal arteriogram in no way disproves the diagnosis. There are, however, many cases reported in which the underlying arterial lesion has been confirmed on an angiogram or a pathological specimen (see Table 8.1). The vessels may indeed appear enlarged, for, as occurs everywhere in the body, the first response to acute ischaemia is vasodilatation. This is a familiar clinical phenomenon in the circulation to the leg, and has been demonstrated by several authors in the colon.[68, 92]

These points are well brought out by Williams and Wittenberg[107] in a study of 55 patients in whom the diagnosis of ischaemic colitis could confidently be made on clinical and radiological grounds. They emphasize that fine vessel angiography gives a better idea of the volume of blood within a vascular bed than the flow taking place through it, and note that in 5 of their 11 patients who were submitted to detailed angiography, the distal vascular bed appeared expanded. Williams and Wittenberg question whether the pathogenesis of spontaneously occurring 'ischaemic colitis' in fact includes ischaemia. Clearly, it is impossible to prove a negative, and, in the absence of a method of directly measuring blood flow in the wall of the living human colon, the question must remain valid. Furthermore, in the non-occlusive cases, the actual time during which blood flow to the colon falls off may in fact be quite brief, occurring perhaps during a transient episode of low cardiac output, so that the opportunity for making instrumental measurements at this point may never arrive. The consequences of vascular impairment in the colon are abundantly documented, and when these features are seen in a patient the simplest

* See References 3, 10, 12, 16, 18, 22, 23, 29, 32, 35, 36, 44, 51, 75, 81, 83, 88, 95, 106, 107, 108.

explanation for them is that of ischaemia, even in the absence of a positive angiogram. This is the hypothesis which, at the time of writing, best fits the facts, and though of course it may be disproved in the future, no rival to it has yet appeared. Ischaemic colitis is such a well known and useful clinical concept that the term has become embedded in the clinical literature, and there seems very little reason to doubt its rightful place.

Classification of ischaemic colitis

Our original description of ischaemic colitis[65] described three forms of the disease graded according to severity. These were as follows.

1. Gangrene of the colon

This group included cases previously labelled 'ischaemic infarction',[58, 85, 101] 'necrotizing colitis',[40] 'ischaemic enterocolitis' and 'gangrene'.[57, 103] These patients presented with an acute abdominal catastrophe, usually undiagnosed before operation, and carrying a very high mortality.

2. Ischaemic stricture

These cases had previously been described 'as regional colitis',[11] 'stenosis',[20, 71] 'benign stricture',[9] 'acute segmental colitis',[49] 'infarction'[19, 26, 43, 64, 97] and 'fibrosis'.[37] They represented an intermediate state of affairs whereby the fall in arterial blood supply to the colon was insufficient to lead to full-thickness necrosis and gangrene, but caused damage to the more specialized and oxygen-demanding layers of the gut, namely the mucosa and the submucosa. The result was the formation of a fibrous stricture.

3. Transient ischaemic colitis

In these cases, which had previously been described as 'reversible vascular occlusion',[8, 12, 18, 25] a relatively minor episode of ischaemia brought about a transient inflammation in the colon which resolved promptly and was followed by complete clinical and radiological recovery.

Though useful at the time, this classification must now be considered obsolete. De Dombal *et al.*,[22] in a thoughtful paper based on a single case report, pointed out that the clinician needed a concept which he could apply at the time the patient presented, and that a grouping which had been drawn up on the basis of retrospective evidence was of little practical use. They suggested that a more rewarding way of looking at the problem would be to classify the patients into two groups; namely, those who respond immediately and obviously to supportive and antibiotic therapy, and those who do not. In this way it should be possible to separate those who have, or may develop, gangrene, from the others who may be expected to recover without surgery. There have been several confirmatory studies since along the same lines,[35, 47, 55, 89] and the subject has recently been reviewed very thoroughly by Williams and Wittenberg[107] who suggest that only two groups are needed, namely those with severe and those with mild disease. They point out that the later development of a stricture is difficult to forecast on the initial clinical presentation, and furthermore that there is no particular point in so doing because not all strictures need surgery.

The precise indications for surgical treatment, based on our own and others' experience, are described in detail below.

Gangrene of the colon

Clinical picture

The patient is characteristically middle-aged or elderly and has a background of degenerative cardiovascular disease such as hypertension, episodes of left ventricular failure and myocardial infarction. He is characteristically under treatment with digitalis, diuretics and potassium supplements. There is no pre-existing history of bowel disturbance and the onset of the present illness is sudden and dramatic, with severe generalized abdominal pain, colicky at first but rapidly becoming diffuse and constant. Almost all patients vomit early in the course of the illness, and diarrhoea is a very frequent feature, although bleeding is unusual.

Over the course of the next few hours this clinical picture gives way to one of progressive abdominal distension, accompanied by thirst, restlessness, air-hunger, and all the symptoms of peripheral circulatory collapse.

Due to the obvious severity of the illness, early medical attention is sought. It is obvious from the most superficial examination that the patient is gravely, even desperately, ill. He is typically pale, sweating and dyspnoeic, with tachycardia and arterial hypotension. The central venous pressure is low.

Examination of the abdomen reveals the signs of a widespread peritonitis with diffuse tenderness, rigidity and absent bowel sounds.

This condition is virtually impossible to diagnose on the clinical picture alone. I have never succeeded in doing so myself, and I have not encountered a single case report among the many in the literature where the diagnosis has been made. The usual clinical impression is of a mesenteric embolus, peritonitis secondary to rupture of the hollow viscus, acute strangulation obstruction, or fulminating pancreatitis.

X-ray appearances

In the very early stages of the illness, the plain film of the abdomen will be normal. After a few hours, the prominent feature is progressive in dilatation of the large[69, 90] and, later, the small bowel, suggesting toxic megacolon or volvulus. A barium enema is clearly inappropriate because of the severity of the illness, and the question of emergency aortography has been discussed above in connection with intestinal failure. The only positive advantage to be gained by aortography is to exclude the possibility of a mesenteric embolus. The abdominal signs are such, however, that no surgeon in his right mind would be dissuaded, by the demonstration of a normal angiogram, from immediate exploration.

Laboratory findings

As in all other forms of acute intestinal ischaemia, early leucocytosis is the rule. There is progressive haemoconcentration with a rise in haematocrit and increase in blood viscosity, accompanied by metabolic acidosis with elevated blood urea and potassium. The serum enzymes follow no very consistent pattern, but changes in transaminase, amylase and lactic dehydrogenase levels may occur, as in other forms of acute abdominal disease. In particular, the intestinal isoenzyme of alkaline phosphatase, which on theoretical grounds might be expected to show considerable rise, has in our experience usually been normal.

Management

This comprises two phases, namely resuscitation and operation (Fig. 8.4).

The first phase of treatment is carried out along the standard lines for correcting the metabolic abnormalities of any patient suffering from a severe intra-abdominal catastrophe. One cannot describe this treatment as specific for colonic gangrene, because the diagnosis has not been made. The clinician is simply presented with a collapsed and dehydrated elderly patient with poor myocardial reserve and signs of peritonitis. The first essential, clearly, is to replenish the circulating volume by local administration of crystalloid (Ringer-lactate or Hartman's) solution and colloid (plasma or low or medium molecular weight dextran), so as to bring down the haematocrit and raise the central venous pressure. Oxygen is given by mask, a nasogastric tube passed and the stomach evacuated, an analgesic premedication given, and preparation is made for immediate emergency exploration of the abdomen.

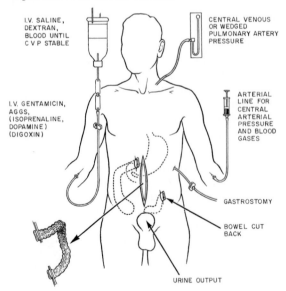

Fig. 8.4. Management of a case of colonic gangrene.

The use of specific pharmacological agents, though logical, has not been reported in clinical series. These would include α-blocking agents such as phenoxybenzamine and β-stimulators such as isoprenaline (both of which promote flow in the mesenteric circulation (see Chapter 3)) and polyvalent anti-gas-gangrene serum (AGGS), to combat the effects of the Clostridia which are known to be important pathogens in certain cases (Fig. 8.4).

Operative technique

In the case of unexplained peritonitis, most surgeons will have opened the abdomen via a small right 'non-committal' paramedian incision, which can be extended upwards and downwards according to what is found. In this instance, it will be immediately obvious on opening the peritoneum that a length of colon (and indeed sometimes of small bowel) has undergone ischaemic necrosis. The appearance of the bowel varies from puce through purple to black and even on occasions dark green, and the length involved may extend for any distance between the rectosigmoid and the caecum. It is, however, unusual to find involvement below the distal pelvic colon. The incision is now enlarged and a quick check made of the peritoneal contents, to exclude any other abnormality. The mesenteric vessels are then inspected and palpated, and are almost invariably found to be patent and pulsatile, up to the margin of the colon. Except in those cases which follow accidental or surgical trauma, colonic gangrene is usually of the non-occlusive variety.

The affected bowel is mobilized in the usual way, by division of the peritoneum on its lateral aspect, but must be handled with great gentleness to avoid tearing its fragile wall and producing massive peritoneal contamination. The vessels at the base of the mesentery are ligated and a length of colon resected between non-crushing clamps, well wide of the abnormal area. The mucosa is then inspected carefully, and the clamps released, in order to confirm that there is pulsatile arterial bleeding from the cut ends. Usually, the mucosal damage is considerably more extensive than would have been suspected from outside, and in this case it is necessary to cut the bowel back still further, in order to be certain of having removed all ischaemic tissue.

No attempt is made to achieve a primary anastomosis. The proximal end of the bowel is exteriorized in any convenient position on the abdominal wall, and the distal end either brought out in the same way or closed and dropped back, according to the length and position of the bowel affected. The peritoneal cavity is then washed out with saline, and the wound closed with appropriate drainage. It is our own practice to insert a gastrostomy tube (Fig. 8.4) for postoperative gastrointestinal decompression; others may prefer the use of a conventional nasogastric tube.

Post-operative management

It is assumed that the patient will be cared for in an intensive therapy unit, along the standard lines. The main complications to be watched for are as follows:

1. Sputum retention leading to pulmonary atelectasis.

2. Exacerbation of pre-existing cardiac problems, including transient arrhythmias, left ventricular failure, angina and myocardial infarction.

3. Cerebral underperfusion, causing confusion and transient focal neurological signs.

4. Venous thrombosis in the lower limbs, with pulmonary embolization.

5. Renal ischaemia with tubular necrosis and oliguria, sometimes complicated by hypercatabolic renal failure.

Apart from these general problems which complicate any type of major surgery in the elderly patient, the most important specific complication is extended gut necrosis. When this occurs, it is almost invariably fatal, but, as explained, its incidence can be minimized by suitably planned resection of the damaged bowel.

Prognosis and mortality

It is generally agreed that gangrene of the colon carries a very high mortality, which is scarcely surprising in that this obviously dangerous condition is prone to occur in people who are already the subjects of degenerative cardiovascular disease. None the less, the figures are skewed by the fact that the diagnosis is usually made only at a late stage in the operation, or at autopsy.[59] Given modern methods of preoperative resuscitation, followed by application of well tried surgical principles, there is no reason why this condition, *per se*, should carry a particularly high death rate. Metabolic disturbances are common to all manner of acute abdominal disease, and the surgery of the acute abdomen, aided as it is by efficient muscular relaxation and supplementary oxygen, fluid and antibiotic therapy, has now lost much of its dangers.

Ischaemic colitis

Terminology

By 'ischaemic colitis' we now mean the non-gangrenous form of the disease, which may vary from a transient episode of inflammation to massive fibrous stricture of the bowel causing complete obstruction.

Clinical picture

This is a disease of the middle-aged and elderly, as would be expected in any condition whose causation is diminished arterial blood supply. Figure 8.5 shows the age incidence of 122 patients described by our group in 1973.[63]

There is usually a background of ischaemic heart disease or peripheral arterial insufficiency, collagen disorder or local colon pathology.

The typical presentation is of acute pain in the left iliac fossa, early nausea and vomiting. This is followed by the passage of one or two loose motions which characteristically contain dark blood and clots.

On examination, the patient does not appear grossly ill nor shocked,

ISCHAEMIC DISEASE OF THE COLON

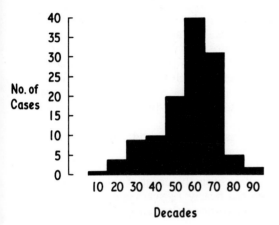

Fig. 8.5. Age incidence of ischaemic colitis (122 cases).

although the temperature and pulse are raised. The constant abdominal finding is of extreme tenderness in the left iliac fossa and in the pelvis, with dark blood on the fingerstall following rectal examination.

Endoscopy

Conventional rigid sigmoidoscopy does not usually bring the lesion into view as the area affected lies above the reach of the instrument. However, there are a few reports in the literature[14, 15] where the dignosis has been made by this means. The appearances described are of irregular heaped-up bluish purple mucosa, with oedema and contact bleeding. They closely resemble the changes found in the colon of the experimental animal, following vascular ligation. Clearly, colonoscopy is likely to prove an extremely useful diagnostic method in the early diagnosis of the disease. As yet, insufficient experience has accumulated to enable any useful comment to be made as to its use, but at the same time no complications or disasters have been reported.

Investigations

Laboratory studies give rather non-specific results. There is almost invariably a polymorph leucocytosis, of 15,000 upwards, and the serum enzymes may be raised in a rather inconsistent fashion.

Plain x-ray will on occasion delineate an area of large bowel whose intraluminal gas shadow demonstrates 'thumb-printing' (see Fig. 8.6). At a later stage in the disease there may be signs of small bowel obstruction, with dilatation of the ileum and fluid levels.

The question of *angiography* remains controversial. While there are many reports in the literature of angiographically demonstrated lesions, non-occlusive disease appears to be more frequent, so that a negative angiogram does not exclude the diagnosis. It is certainly not required as a routine examination in every case.[69, 96, 108]

Barium studies

The barium enema has undoubtedly been the most useful diagnostic tool in the diagnosis of ischaemic colitis. The appearances have been studied in detail by many radiologists, and are now well established.[27, 96, 99, 108]

Unless the patient is very ill, the bowel is prepared by a standard technique such as an oxyphenisatin enema, to clear it of faeces. The colon is filled with barium under the image intensifier, and the usual series of posteroanterior and oblique views taken, followed by postevacuation and air insufflation films.

The changes seen on the contrast enema depend, naturally, upon the timing of the examination. They are as follows.

1. *Thumb-printing* is the earliest change seen on the barium enema, and has been observed as early as 3 days after the onset of the symptoms.[96, 108] The term was originally suggested nearly 14 years ago by Boley and his group[8] and in spite of other suggestions ('pseudopolyposis', 'polypoid

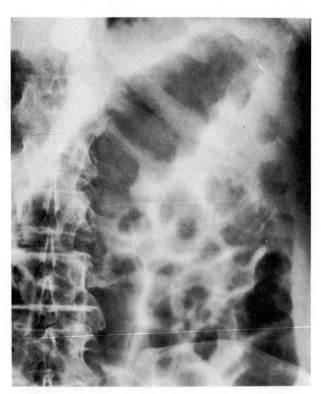

Fig. 8.6. Plain x-ray in ischaemic colitis, showing thumb-printing. (By courtesy of Dr Michael Lea Thomas.)

change', 'scalloping') has stood the test of time. It is illustrated in Figs. 8.6 and 8.7, and can also be seen experimentally (Chapter 4). The sign consists in a series of blunt semi-opaque projections into the intestinal lumen, with a margin of half-shadowing, and once experienced is quite unmistakable. Correlation with the endoscopic findings in the experimental animal leaves little doubt that the large thumb-prints are due to submucosal oedema and haemorrhage. Although they are seen most frequently in the region of the splenic flexure, they may occur anywhere from caecum to pelvi-rectal junction.

Thumb-printing is an early change, and has been recorded as disappearing at an interval as short as 48 hours. It may, however, persist for several weeks.[99]

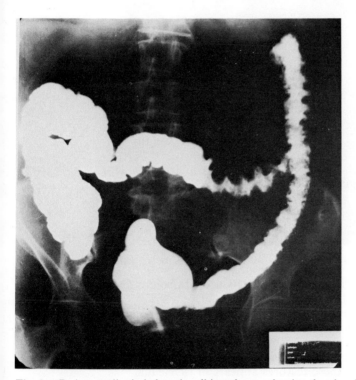

Fig. 8.7. Barium studies in ischaemic colitis early case showing thumb-printing.

2. *Mucosal irregularity.* During the days or weeks following the onset of the illness, the radiological appearances may alter in two directions. In many instances, the original thumb-printing clears completely, and the outline of the bowel returns to normal (see Fig. 8.11). However, depending on the degree of vascular insult, the appearance may progress to the next phase, namely that of *mucosal ulceration and irregularity* (Figs. 8.8–8.11). The ulcers are of varying size and depth and are quite irregular in their disposition around the circumference of the bowel. A barium enema taken at this stage may produce changes reminiscent of those of ulcerative colitis,

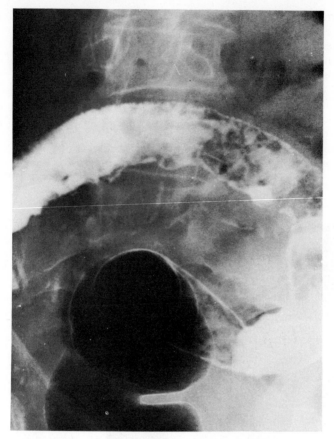

Fig. 8.8. Barium studies in ischaemic colitis: appearances 10 days following aortic resection.

and confusion with the transmural fissures of Crohn's disease has also been recorded.

However, in ulcerative colitis there is invariably rectal involvement, with loss of haustration and a uniform abolition of mucosal pattern. In Crohn's disease one sees deep transmural fissures giving the 'rose thorn' appearance, and the lesions are characteristically separated by areas of normal bowel. None of these features appears in ischaemia.

3. Once again, the changes can be reversible or progress to irreversibility. In the latter event, the next phase of radiological change is stricture formation, which appears on the radiograph as *tubular narrowing*, with or without *sacculation* on the antimesenteric aspect of the bowel. When correlated with the pathological appearances, it is found that tubular narrowing is due to heavy and fairly symmetrical deposition of fibrous tissues throughout the submucosa, whereas sacculation occurs when the fibrous tissue is deposited in a more uneven, but none the less annular, fashion. Sacculation is, in fact, rather unusual, but when seen, coupled with the clinical history, is virtually pathognomic of late-stage ischaemia. Once again, the common location is around the splenic flexure. This replacement of the specialized

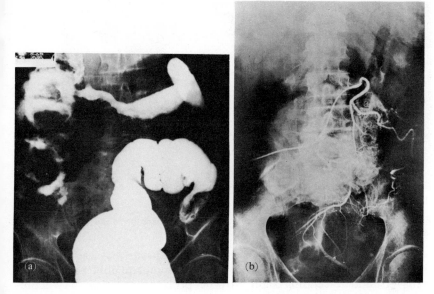

Fig. 8.9. Barium studies in ischaemic colitis: late case showing ulceration and narrowing. (a) Barium study; (b) selective angiogram, showing abnormal segment outlined by gas, and without arterial circulation.

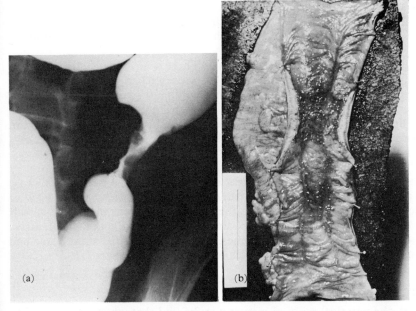

Fig. 8.10. Barium studies in ischaemic colitis: a localized ischaemic stricture. (a) Barium study (by courtesy of Dr Michael Lea Thomas); (b) the operative specimen.

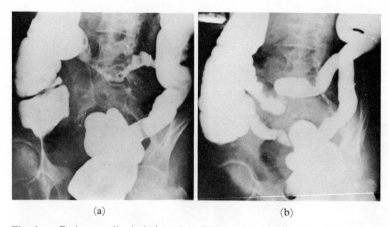

(a)   (b)

Fig. 8.11. Barium studies in ischaemic colitis: segmental infarction of the transverse colon. (a) Initial appearance; (b) 4 months later.

layers of the submucosa by contracting fibrous tissue may vary in extent from a few centimetres in the splenic area to complete obliteration of the transverse and descending colon. No other process than ischaemia will produce such dramatic contraction (or even at times obliteration) of the colonic lumen over a period of a few weeks.

On occasion the narrowing occurs over a very limited segment of the bowel. This appearance gives rise to diagnostic difficulty because any localized stricture must of course be regarded as malignant, until proven otherwise. A differentiating feature here is the appearance which Lea Thomas has termed 'funnelling'[99] (see Fig. 8.10), which presents a smooth graduated beginning and end to the stricture, quite different from the irregular 'shoulders' which one associates with an ulcerating malignant tumour.

The timing of the barium enema.   There is no evidence that an early barium enema has ever harmed a patient with ischaemic colitis. Obviously, when the colon is gangrenous, such an examination would be very dangerous, but this is not a practical clinical situation. In the absence of immediate facilities for colonoscopy, there is no question but that an early barium enema is a most valuable and safe adjunct to the management of any case of acute colonic inflammation.

Rectal involvement.   Our initial impression was that ischaemic disease never attacked the rectum. This finding was not unexpected in view of the very rich collateral supply to the lower bowel from the pelvic vessels (see Chapter 2). Later experience showed that, in patients with occlusive disease of the lower aortic branches, ischaemic proctitis could occur and cause confusion with other causes of rectal inflammation.[30, 51, 84]

Management

From the practical point of view it may be said that when the patient has been assessed as has been described it then becomes possible to draw a fairly accurate distinction between what is *probably* ischaemic colitis, where continued observation and further assessment is justified, and what is *probably* some form of purulent peritonitis or haemorrhagic condition, where immediate exploration of the abdomen is mandatory. The crucial diagnostic step is to obtain a barium enema at the earliest possible opportunity, because the appearances are so characteristic.

Once the diagnosis has been established, treatment should in almost every case be expectant. That is to say, the patient is rested in bed, given an intravenous or fluid regimen, according to the degree of peritoneal irritation, and monitored by daily leucocyte counts and haematocrit readings. It is our practice to administer systemic ampicillin, rather on *a priori* grounds, as it has been established that systemic antibiotics mitigate the effect of colonic ischaemia in the experimental laboratory (see Chapter 4), but it must be admitted that the logic behind this therapy is quite uncontrolled, and it may in fact be unnecessary. Anticoagulants, here as in other situations of acute arterial occlusion, are unlikely to influence the pathological process, and are not indicated. Indeed, it is possible that their use might exacerbate bleeding in what is, after all, a haemorrhagic infarct. Needless to say, there is no place whatever for the use of corticosteroids.

On this expectant regimen, there are three possible sequelae:[63]

1. Progression to gangrene
2. Resolution (transient ischaemic colitis)
3. Stricture formation

For a patient with acute non-gangrenous ischaemic colitis to develop gangrene of the colon is, fortunately, extremely rare.[71] In our personal series[63] it occurred only twice in 122 cases. The usual course of events is for the pain, bleeding and diarrhoea to settle rapidly over the course of a few days, or perhaps a week or two, and for a subsequent barium enema to show a normal colon, or one with minimal involvement (see Fig. 8.11). Sometimes, probably in about one-third of all cases, a fibrous stricture develops, but this is frequently quite asymptomatic and does not in itself require treatment.

Not every patient presents as an emergency in the early stage of the disease. It is quite common for a patient to arrive with a 3 or 4 weeks' history of large bowel symptoms, and for the barium enema then to show mucosal narrowing and ulceration, or stricture formation. The history in these cases being typical, one surmises that, had an opportunity arisen of seeing the patient earlier, the characteristic changes of 'thumb-printing' would have been observed, but of course there is no objective certainty of this. In any event, surgical treatment is not urgent, and plenty of time should be allowed for the symptoms to subside, with repeated endoscopy and barium examination.

Indications for surgery

These are:

1. Gangrene (rare)
2. Persistent bleeding due to deep ulceration

3. Obstructive symptoms
4. The possibility of malignancy

In our series of 58 strictures,[63] 49 patients underwent resection, of whom 4 died. Of the remaining 9 patients treated conservatively, 1 died from a cerebrovascular accident. However, it should be borne in mind that this series includes a number of cases seen in the early 1960s, when ischaemic colitis was much less well recognized, and many of these patients would not be operated upon today. It must be stressed, as has been pointed out by Williams and his colleagues,[106, 107] that a stricture is not, *per se*, an indication for surgery, and it is incorrect to correlate the occurrence of a stricture with the severe form of disease which carries a poor prognosis. The only strictures which require operation are those which distress by persistent bleeding, cramps, diarrhoea or other obstructive symptoms, or which could be neoplastic.

Operative treatment

Surgical resection of an ischaemic stricture of the colon does not differ in any important respect from operations carried out for cancer or diverticular disease. The area most frequently affected is the splenic flexure, so that it is our practice to carry out the operation in the Lloyd-Davies position, as for an abdominoperineal excision of the rectum, which provides access to the perineum. A long left paramedian incision is made and the splenic flexure mobilized. Obviously, especial care should be taken over the vascularity of the resected ends, but provided that the mucosa is pink and healthy with pulsatile vessels up to its margins, and that the anastomosis is made without tension, no particular difficulty is encountered and the incidence of anastomotic breakdown is not high.

Pathology of ischaemic colitis

For detailed accounts of the pathological appearances the reader is referred to the writings of Morson.[66, 78] The main characteristics are as follows.

Gross appearances

In *gangrene of the colon* (Fig. 8.12) the bowel appears black or even green, dilated and thinned, with absent mucosa, gross ulceration and even on occasion frank perforation. Except in those cases which are known to follow a vascular injury or operation, it is unusual to find major occlusions of the supplying vessels.

In *non-gangrenous ischaemic colitis* the colon appears thickened, rigid and not unlike the picturesquely described 'eel in rigor mortis', in connection with large bowel Crohn's disease. The exact appearances will depend on at which stage in the illness the specimen was taken. Early change (coinciding with the radiological appearance of thumb-printing) will appear as coarse, 'cobble-stoning' of the mucosa, with linear ulceration and surface haemorrhage. The length of bowel involved may be from 5 to 25 cm, and on occasion can involve the entire colon. Where there is a limited stricture,

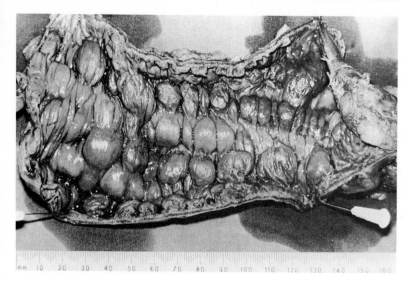

Fig. 8.12. Gangrene of the colon.

the gross appearance is quite different from that of a carcinoma, in that the mucosa is ulcerated in a shallow pattern, and there is a heavy deposition of thick white fibrous tissue in the submucosa, easily appreciated by the naked eye (Fig. 8.13). Frequently there is an associated thickening of the serosal coats, with condensation of the surrounding fatty tissue, namely in the appendices epiploicae, and in the mesentery.

Microscopic appearances

In *gangrene of the colon* the appearances are very much the same as those shown in Figs. 4.5 and 4.6) with respect to the terminal stages of acute

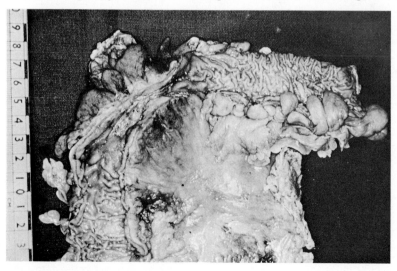

Fig. 8.13. Ischaemic stricture of the colon.

small bowel ischaemia. If the mucosa has sloughed, there is an intense infiltration of inflammatory cells into the deeper layers, and the muscle layers show severe destruction of their fibres, with vacuolation of the cytoplasm and pyknosis of the nuclei.

In *non-gangrenous ischaemic colitis* there is full-thickness loss of mucosa in the ulcerated areas, whose base is composed of congested granulation tissue. There may be some epithelial regeneration at the edges. Between the ulcers, the mucosa shows patchy atrophy and irregularity, with splaying of the muscle fibres of the muscularis mucosae. The most striking changes are found in the submucosal layers (Fig. 8.14) which are greatly thickened and filled with proliferating fibroblasts, oedema and inflammatory cells including lymphocytes, eosinophils and plasma cells. A characteristic finding which is common both to the clinical and the experimentally produced specimens, is the presence of haemosiderin-laden

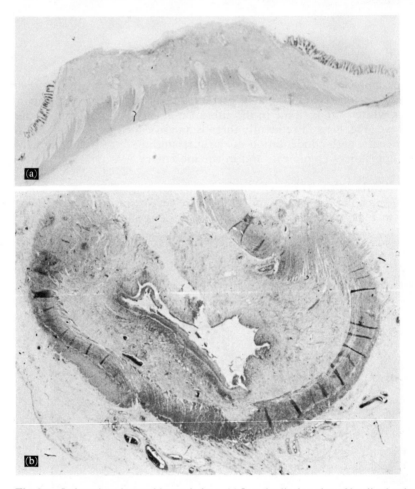

Fig. 8.14. Ischaemic stricture: histopathology. (a) Longitudinal section of localized stricture; (b) transverse section of extensive stricture.

macrophages, much as are found in a resolving myocardial infarct. For this reason, it is a wise policy to examine with Perls' Prussian blue method any resected specimen of colon whose pathological appearances are not wholly typical (Fig. 8.15).

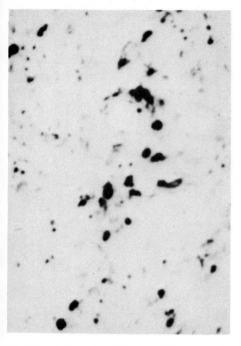

Fig. 8.15. Ischaemic colitis: iron-laden macrophages in the submucosa.

Differential diagnosis

In a typical case presenting as an emergency the diagnosis should be fairly straightforward, particularly if there is associated rectal bleeding. The main conditions with which it is to be confused are as follows:

1. Infective gastroenteritis.
2. Acute diverticular disease, including ruptured pericolic abscess, and perforation of the colon.
3. Acute large bowel Crohn's disease, or exacerbation of chronic inflammatory disease.
4. Perforation of a hollow viscus such as the stomach, or duodenum with peritonitis tracking down the left side of the abdomen.
5. Acute pancreatitis.
6. Left-sided renal colic.
7. Leaking abdominal aortic aneurysm.

It is quite likely that many episodes of abdominal pain and diarrhoea, particularly in the older age groups, which are diagnosed as gastroenteritis or diverticular disease are in fact transient ischaemic episodes. There is

Table 8.2 Clinical differential diagnosis of ischaemic colitis

	Ulcerative colitis	Crohn's disease	Ischaemic colitis
Age at onset	10–30	30–40	60+
Course	Chronic, relapsing; tendency to malignancy	Chronic	Acute episodes
Associated conditions	Iritis, arthritis, pyodermia	Megaloblastic anaemia, fistulae	Arterial disease, collagen disease, diabetes
Site	Left-sided or total, rectum always involved	Anywhere, rectum usually involved	Splenic flexure, rectum almost never involved
Radiology	Shortening, loss of haustration	Fissures, skip areas	Polypoid change, tubular narrowing, sacculation

Table 8.3 Pathological diagnosis of ischaemic colitis

	Ischaemic colitis	Crohn's disease	Ulcerative colitis
Depth of inflammation	Transmural	Transmural	Mucosal submucosal (except in fulminating colitis)
Submucosa	Widened	Widened	Normal width or reduced
Focal aggregates of lymphocytes	Absent or very few	Always (often transmural)	Sometimes (restricted to mucosa and submucosa)

Crypt abscesses	Absent	Few	Very common
Goblet-cell population of mucosa	Reduced (acute phase). Normal (ischaemic stricture)	Normal or slight reduction	Much reduced in active disease
Paneth cell metaplasia	Uncommon	Uncommon	Common
Sarcoid granulomas	Absent	Present about 60%	Absent
Fissuring	Absent	Common	Absent
Precancerous epithelial changes	No	No	Yes
Mucosal necrosis	Yes (acute phase)	No	No
Intravascular platelet thrombi	Yes (acute phase)	No	No
Submucosal oedema	Yes (acute phase)	Yes	Usually absent
Vascularity	Yes (acute phase)	Not prominent	Very prominent, particularly in active disease
Fibrosis	Usually very pronounced (ischaemic stricture)	Moderate or absent	None
Secondary vasculitis	Yes	Rare	Rare
Haemosiderin-laden macrophages	Yes	No	No
Hyalinization of connective tissue in submucosa	Yes	Never	No
Muscle necrosis	Common	Never	Only in toxic megacolon
Muscle fibrosis	Common	Never	Never

Reproduced from *Vascular Disorders of the Intestine* (1971; Ed. by S. J. Boley), by kind permission of Dr B. C. Morson and the publishers, Appleton-Century-Crofts, New York.

no way to prove this point, but common sense would suggest that such is the case. The feature which distinguishes ischaemia from other conditions is the presence of the characteristic dark rectal bleeding, though this occurs only in some two-thirds of cases.[63] Often, the diagnosis is not made immediately, but comes to light only with the barium enema.

When seen later in the course of the illness, the condition may closely resemble Crohn's disease or ulcerative colitis. The main distinguishing features are set out in Tables 8.2 and 8.3. The most important of these are the characteristic age range of the patients, the association with degenerative cardiovascular disease, and the distinctive radiological and pathological appearances.

Summary and conclusions

Ischaemic colitis is now a well recognized and established clinical condition, which may occur spontaneously or following interference with the vasculature of the colon. Two quite distinct forms of the illness occur, and it is rare, though not unknown, for one to progress to the other. In the first place there is a severe form of colitis due to full-thickness necrosis of the colonic wall, which presents as an abdominal catastrophe, requires urgent excisional surgery and carries a high mortality. The milder form of the illness presents as an acute left-sided peritonitis, usually associated with diarrhoea and rectal bleeding, and can safely be treated expectantly. About half the patients managed in this way will form a fibrous stricture in the colon, but only a minority of these develop symptoms which are bad enough to warrant operation.

References

1   Ambruoso, V. N. and Ferrari, F. (1967). Massive gangrene of the colon due to distal obstruction. *Surgery* **61**: 228–230.
2   Ault, G. W., Castro, A. F. and Smith, R. S. (1952). Clinical study of ligation of the inferior mesenteric artery in left colon resections. *Surgery, Gynecology and Obstetrics* **94**: 223–228.
3   Balslev, I., Jensen, H., Norgaard, F. and Poll, P. (1970). Ischaemic colitis. *Acta Chirurgica Scandinavica* **136**: 235–242.
4   Bernstein, W. C. and Bernstein, E. F. (1963). Ischemic ulcerative colitis following mesenteric arterial ligation. *Diseases of the Colon and Rectum* **6**: 54–61.
5   Bicks, R. O., Bale, G. F., Howard, H. and McBurney, R. F. (1968). Acute and delayed colon ischemia after resection of aortic aneurysm. *Archives of Internal Medicine* **122**: 249–253.
6   Birnbaum, W., Rudy, L. and Wylie, E. J. (1964). Colonic and rectal ischemia following aortic aneurysmectomy. *Diseases of the Colon and Rectum* **7**: 293–302.
7   Boley, S. J. and Schwartz, S. S. (1971). Colitis complicating carcinoma of the colon. In: *Vascular Disorders of the Intestine*, pp. 631–642. Ed. by S. J. Boley. New York and London, Appleton-Century-Crofts.
8   Boley, S. J., Schwartz, S., Lash, J. and Sternhill, V. (1963). Reversible vascular occlusion of the colon. *Surgery, Gynecology and Obstetrics* **116**: 53–60.

9 Boreham, P. (1957). Benign strictures of the colon. *Proceedings of the Royal Society of Medicine* **50**: 601–604.

10 Brown, A. R. (1968). Diagnosis and management of non-gangrenous ischaemic colitis. *Gut* **9**: 737–739.

11 Brownlee, T. J. (1951). Regional colitis as an acute abdominal emergency. *British Journal of Surgery* **38**: 507–509.

12 Byrd, B. F., Sawyers, J. L., Bomar, R. L. and Klatte, E. C. (1968). Reversible vascular occlusion of the colon: recognition and management. *Annals of Surgery* **167**: 901–908.

13 Cannon, J. A. (1955). Discussion. *American Journal of Surgery* **90**: 315.

14 Carter, R., Vannix, R., Hinshaw, D. B. and Stafford, C. E. (1959). Inferior mesenteric vascular occlusion—sigmoidoscopic diagnosis. *Surgery* **46**: 845–846.

15 Carter, R., Vannix, R., Hinshaw, D. B. and Stafford, C. E. (1959). Acute inferior mesenteric vascular occlusion: a surgical syndrome. *American Journal of Surgery* **98**: 271–275.

16 Castelli, M. F., Qizilbach, A. H., Salem, S. and Fyshe, T. G. (1974). Ischaemic bowel disease. *Canadian Medical Association Journal* **111**: 935–941.

17 Clark, A. W., Lloyd-Mostyn, R. H. and Sadler, M. R. de C. (1972). Ischaemic colitis in young adults. *British Medical Journal* **4**: 70–72.

18 Coligado, E. Y. and Fleshler, B. (1967). Reversible vascular occlusion of the colon. *Radiology* **89**: 432–434.

19 Cooling, C. I. and Protheroe, R. H. B. (1958). Infarction of the colon. *Postgraduate Medical Journal* **34**: 494–497.

20 Corbett, R. (1957). Stenosed segment of descending colon associated with trauma. *Proceedings of the Royal Society of Medicine* **50**: 271–272.

21 Cotton, P. B. and Thomas, M. L. (1971). Ischaemic colitis and the contraceptive pill. *British Medical Journal* **3**: 27–29.

22 de Dombal, F. T., Fierher, D. M. and Harris, R. S. (1969). Early diagnosis of ischaemic colitis. *Gut* **10**: 131–134.

23 Deloyers, L. (1970). Colite ischémique chez un jeune homme—forme sténosante rectosigmoidienne. *Acta Gastro-enterologica Belgica* **33**: 800–803.

24 Descotes, J., Bouchet, A., Sisteron, A. and George, P. (1963). La Réimplantation de l'artère mésenterique supérieur dans le traitement de l'insuffisance artérielle intestinale. *Lyon Chirurgical* **59**: 5–8.

25 Dunbar, J. D. (1966). Reversible cecal infarction—a case report with angiographic follow-up study. *American Journal of Surgery* **112**: 447–449.

26 Engelhardt, J. E. and Jacobson, G. (1956). Infarction of colon demonstrated by barium enema. *Radiology* **67**: 573–574.

27 Farman, J. (1971). The radiologic features of colonic vascular disease. In: *Vascular Disorders of the Intestine*, pp. 229–242. Ed by S. J. Boley. New York and London, Appleton-Century-Crofts.

28 Feller, E., Rickert, R. and Spiro, H. M. (1971). Small vessel disease of the gut. In: *Vascular Disorders of the Intestine*, pp. 483–509. Ed. by S. J. Boley. New York and London, Appleton-Century-Crofts.

29 Gambee, L. P. (1937). Occlusion of the inferior mesenteric vessels. *Western Journal of Surgery* **45**: 105–108.

30 Ganchrow, M. I., Clark, J. F. and Ferguson, J. A. (1970). Ischemic proctitis with obliterative vascular change. *Diseases of the Colon and Rectum* **13**: 470–471.

31 Gelfand, M. D. (1972). Ischemic colitis associated with a depot synthetic progestogen. *American Journal of Digestive Diseases* **17**: 275–277.

32 Gibson, W. E., Pearce, G. W. and Creech, O. (1969). Infarction of the left colon due to primary vascular occlusion. *Disorders of the Colon and Rectum* **12**: 323–326.

33   Goligher, J. C. (1954). The adequacy of the marginal blood supply to the left colon after high ligation of the inferior mesenteric artery during excision of the rectum. *British Journal of Surgery* **41**: 351–358.

34   Gonzalez, L. L. and Jaffe, M. S. (1966). Mesenteric arterial insufficiency following abdominal aortic resection. *Archives of Surgery* **93**: 10–20.

35   Haddad, H. (1974). Clinical features of ischemic bowel disease. *Canadian Journal of Surgery* **17**: 434–446.

36   Hammelbo, S., Kavlie, H., Gjone, E. and Øystese, B. (1967). Ischemisk colitt. *Nordisk Medicin* **77**: 805–807.

37   Hannan, J. R., Jackson, B. P. and Pipik, P. (1964). Fibrosis and stenosis of the descending colon following occlusion of the inferior mesenteric artery. *American Journal of Roentgenology* **91**: 826–832.

38   Harrison, A. W. and Croal, A. E. (1962). Left colon ischaemia following occlusion or ligation of the superior mesenteric artery. *Canadian Journal of Surgery* **5**: 293–298.

39   Hartmann, H. A. (1909). Some considerations upon high amputations of the rectum. *Annals of Surgery* **50**: 1091–1097.

40   Heikinnen, E., Laurri, T. K. I. and Huttunen, R. (1974). Necrotizing colitis. *American Journal of Surgery* **128**: 362–367.

41   Herrmann, J. W., Paine, J. R. and Stubbe, N. J. (1965). Acute obstruction with gangrene of the colon secondary to carcinoma of the sigmoid. *Surgery* **57**: 647–650.

42   Huggard, R. and Herstein, A. (1948). Thrombosis of the inferior mesenteric artery. *Canadian Medical Association Journal* **62**: 502–503.

43   Irwin, A. (1965). Partial infarction of the colon due to reversible vascular occlusion. *Clinical Radiology* **16**: 261–263.

44   Jacobs, E. (1970). A propos de deux cas de nécrose étendue de la muqueuse colique. *Acta Gastro-enterologica Belgica* **33**: 804–810.

45   Johnson, W. C. and Nabseth, D. C. (1974). Visceral infarction following aortic surgery. *Annals of Surgery* **180**: 312–318.

46   Joyeux, R., Courty, A., Biscaye, A., Carli, G. and Lisbonne, M. (1950). Une complication grave et inédite de l'aortographie. *Semaine des Hôpitaux de Paris* **26**: 152–156.

47   Kaminski, D. L., Keltner, R. M. and Willman, V. L. (1973). Ischemic colitis. *Archives of Surgery* **106**: 558–563.

48   Kawarada, Y., Satinsky, S. and Matsumoto, T. (1974). Ischemic colitis following rectal prolapse. *Surgery* **76**: 340–343.

49   Kellock, T. D. (1957). Acute segmental ulcerative colitis. *Lancet* **2**: 660–663.

50   Killen, D. A., Sewell, R. and Foster, J. H. (1967). Colonic injury resulting from angiographic contrast media. *American Journal of Surgery* **114**: 904–909.

51   Kilpatrick, Z. M., Farman, J., Yesner, R. and Spiro, H. M. (1968). Ischemic proctitis. *Journal of the American Medical Association* **205**: 74–80.

52   Kilpatrick, Z. M., Silverman, J. F., Betancourt, E., Farman, J. and Lawson, J. P. (1968). Vascular occlusion of the colon and oral contraceptives. *New England Journal of Medicine* **278**: 438–440.

53   Kummel, H. (1899). Uber resektion des Colon descenden und fixation des Colon Transversum in den Analimen. *Archiv für Klinische Chirurgie* **59**: 555–558.

54   Lambana, S., Yamamoto, K., Miyashita, T. and Tsuchiya, K. (1973). Irreversible ischemic colitis caused by stenosis of sigmoid branches, a case report. *Surgery* **74**: 587–592.

55   Larmi, T. K. I., Heikinnen, E. and Huttunen, R. (1975). Ischaemic and necrotizing colitis. *Annales Chirurgiae et Gynaecologiae Fenniae* **64**: 1–3.

56   Lauenstein, C. (1882). Ein unerwartetes Ereignis nach der Pylorusresektion. *Zentralblatt für Chirurgie* **9**: 137–141.

57   Lister, E. and Jungmann, H. (1956). Gangrene of the colon. *British Journal of Radiology* **29**: 341–343.

58   McCort, J. J. (1960). Infarction of the descending colon due to vascular occlusion. *New England Journal of Medicine* **262**: 168–172.

59   McGovern, V. J. and Goulstone, S. G. M. (1965). Ischaemic enterocolitis. *Gut* **6**: 213–220.

60   McKain, J. and Schumacker, H. B. (1958). Ischemia of the left colon associated with abdominal aortic aneurysms and their treatment. *Archives of Surgery* **76**: 355–357.

61   Marcuson, R. W. and Farman, J. (1971). Ischaemic disease of the colon. *Proceedings of the Royal Society of Medicine* **64**: 1080–1083.

62   Marcuson, R. W., Stewart, J. O. and Marston, A. (1972). Experimental venous lesions of the colon. *Gut* **13**: 1–7.

63   Marcuson, R. W. (1972). Ischaemic colitis. *Clinics in Gastroenterology* **1**: 745–765.

64   Marston, A. (1962). Massive infarction of the colon demonstrated radiologically. *British Journal of Surgery* **49**: 609–611.

65   Marston, A., Pheils, M. T., Thomas, M. L. and Morson, B. C. (1966). Ischaemic colitis. *Gut* **7**: 1–10.

66   Marston, A. (1966). Ischaemic disease of the colon. *Proceedings of the Royal Society of Medicine* **59**: 881–883.

67   Marston, A. (1967). Vascular disorders of the colon. *Acta Chirurgica Belgica* **11**: 80–82.

68   Marston, A., Marcuson, R. W., Chapman, M. and Arthur, J. F. (1969) Experimental study of devascularization of the colon. *Gut* **10**: 121–130.

69   Marston, A. (1972). Diagnosis and management of intestinal ischaemia. *Annals of the Royal College of Surgeons* **50**: 29–44.

70   Matthews, J. G. W. and Parks, T. G. (1972). Production of ischaemic colitis experimentally in the dog by vasoconstriction and hypotensive techniques. *Gut* **13**: 323.

71   Mays, E. T. and Noer, R. J. (1966). Colonic stenosis after trauma. *Journal of Trauma* **6**: 316–329.

72   Miller, J. H. and Bennett, R. C. (1968). Ischaemic strictures of the rectosigmoid complicating resections of abdominal aortic aneurysms. *Australia and New Zealand Journal of Surgery* **37**: 345–350.

73   Miller, R. E. and Knox, W. G. (1966). Colon Ischemia following infra renal aortic surgery. *Annals of Surgery* **163**: 639–643.

74   Miller, W. T., Scott, J., Rosato, E. F., Rosato, P. E. and Crow, H. (1970). Ischemic colitis with gangrene. *Radiology* **94**: 291–297.

75   Mitchell, H. G., Coppola, F. S., Desmery, R. and Iotti, R. (1971). Colitis isquémicas. (1971). *Acta Gastroenterologica Latinoamericana* **3**: 61–70.

76   Mogadam, M., Schuman, B. M., Duncan, H. and Patton, R. B. (1969). Necrotizing colitis associated with rheumatoid arthritis. *Gastroenterology* **57**: 168–172.

77   Morgan, C. N. and Griffiths, J. D. (1959). High ligation of the inferior mesenteric artery during operations for carcinoma of the distal colon and rectum. *Surgery, Gynecology and Obstetrics* **108**: 641–650.

78   Morson, B. C. (1972). The pathology of ischaemic colitis. *Clinics in Gastroenterology* **1**: 765–766.

79   Movius, H. (1955). Resection of abdominal aortic aneurysm. *American Journal of Surgery* **90**: 298–305.

80 Neto, J. A. R. and Ribeiro, A. P. (1974). Trombose mesentérica inferior. *Revista da Associaçao Medica Brasileira* **20**: 180–190.

81 O'Connell, T. X., Kadell, B. and Tompkins, R. K. (1976). Ischemia of the colon. *Surgery, Gynecology and Obstetrics* **142**: 337–342.

82 Padhi, R. K. (1960). Fatal infarction of the descending colon after lumbar aortography. *Canadian Medical Association Journal* **82**: 199–201.

83 Parks, T. G. (1972). Ischaemic colitis. *Proceedings of the Royal Society of Medicine* **65**: 784.

84 Parks, T. G., Johnston, C. W., Kennedy, T. L. and Gough, A. D. (1972). Spontaneous ischaemic proctocolitis. *Scandinavian Journal of Gastroenterology* **7**: 241–246.

85 Payan, H., Levine, S., Bronstein, L. and King, E. (1965). Subtotal ischemic infarction of colon simulating ulcerative colitis. *Archives of Pathology* **80**: 530–533.

86 Penn, I. (1970). Major colonic problems in human homotransplant recipients. *Archives of Surgery* **100**: 61–65.

87 Perdue, G. D. and Lowry, K. (1962). Arterial insufficiency to the colon following resection of abdominal aortic aneurysms. *Surgery, Gynecology and Obstetrics* **115**: 39–44.

88 Pheils, M. T. (1969). Ischaemic colitis. *Medical Journal of Australia* **2**: 715–716.

89 Pierce, G. E. and Brockenbrough, E. C. (1970). The spectrum of mesenteric infarction. *American Journal of Surgery* **119**: 233–241.

90 Pope, C. E. and Judd, E. S. (1929). The arterial blood supply of the sigmoid, rectosigmoid and rectum. *Surgical Clinics of North America* **9**: 957–960.

91 Powis, S. J. A., Barnes. A. D., Dawson-Edwards, P. and Thompson, H. (1972). Ileocolonic problems after cadaveric renal transplantation. *British Medical Journal* **1**: 99–101.

92 Reuter, S. R., Kanter, I. E. and Redman, H. C. (1970). Angiography in reversible colonic ischemia. *Radiology* **97**: 371–375.

93 Rosato, E. F., Rosato, F. E., Scott, J., Crow, H. and Miller, W. T. (1969). Ischemic dilatation of the colon. *American Journal of Digestive Diseases* **14**: 922–928.

94 Saegesser, F., Phillips, V. Chapuis, G., and Rausis, C. (1972). Cancers associés à la rectocolite ulcéro-hemorragique et aux autres manifestations inflammatioires ulcéro-hémorragiques du gros intestin. *Schweizerische Rundschau für Medicin* **7**: 200–206.

95 Saegesser, F., Fasel, J. and Rausis, C. (1972). Manifestations inflammatoires ulcéro-hémorragiques du gros intestin. *Schweizer von Medizin* **61**: 191–192.

96 Sherbon, K. J. (1970). Radiology of ischaemic colitis. *Australasian Radiology* **14**: 46–55.

97 Shippey, S. H. and Acker, J. J. (1965). Segmental infarction of the colon demonstrated by selective inferior mesenteric angiography. *American Journal of Surgery* **109**: 671–675.

98 Smith, R. F. and Szilagyi, D. E. (1960). Ischemia of the colon as a complication in the surgery of the abdominal aorta. *Archives of Surgery* **80**: 806–811.

99 Thomas, M. L. (1968). Further observations on ischaemic colitis. *Proceedings of the Royal Society of Medicine* **61**: 341–342.

100 Thomas, M. L. and Wellwood, J. M. (1973). Ischaemic colitis and abdomino-perineal excision of the rectum. *Gut* **14**: 64–67.

101 Thomson, F. B. (1948). Ischemic infarction of the left colon. *Canadian Medical Association Journal* **58**: 183–185.

102 Treves, F. (1898). Idiopathic dilation of the colon. *Lancet* **1**: 276–279.

103 Wald, M. (1964). Gangrene of the distal two thirds of transverse colon, left

colon, rectum and anal canal due to superior mesenteric vascular insufficiency. *Diseases of the Colon and Rectum* **7**: 303–305.

104 Westcott, J. L. (1972). Angiographic demonstration of arterial occlusion in ischemic colitis. *Gastroenterology* **63**: 486–490.

105 Wilder, R. J. and Steichen, F. M. (1960). Necrosis of the entire gastrointestinal tract following translumbar aortography. *Archives of Surgery* **80**: 198–203.

106 Williams, L. F., Bosniak, M. A. and Wittenberg, J. (1969). Ischemic colitis. *American Journal of Surgery* **117**: 254–263.

107 Williams, L. F. and Wittenberg, J. (1975). Ischemic colitis: a useful clinical diagnosis, but is it ischemic? *Annals of Surgery* **182**: 439–448.

108 Wittenberg, J., Athanosoulis, C. A., Williams, L. F., Papedes, S., O'Sullivan, P. and Brown, B. (1975). Ischemic colitis—radiology and pathophysiology. *American Journal of Roentgenology* **123**: 287–299.

109 Young, J. R., Britton, R. E. and de Wolfe, V. G. (1962). Intestinal ischemic necrosis, following abdominal aorta surgery. *Surgery, Gynecology and Obstetrics* **115**: 615–620.

110 Young, J. R., Humphries, A. W., de Wolfe, V. G. and Lefevre, F. A. (1963). Complications of abdominal aortic surgery. Part II. Intestinal ischemia. *Archives of Surgery* **86**: 51–59.

9

Rarities

Arterial trauma

The visceral arteries are among the most deeply placed and inaccessible structures in the body, and lie in close relation to many vital organs. For practical purposes, therefore, injury to them only occurs in association with major and widespread trauma from which the patient often succumbs before reaching hospital. Thus in a recent review of 126 civilian arterial injuries, Bole *et al.*[1] quoted only 1 case each of injury to the hepatic, superior mesenteric and inferior mesenteric arteries. Clearly, however, management of the visceral circulation will be a major preoccupation in repair of injuries of the lower thoracic and upper abdominal aorta, although the arterial trunks themselves may have remained unscathed.

There is very little information on the maximum tolerable period of interruption of the SMA in the healthy young adult, though from animal experiments and from the analogy of mesenteric embolus, some degree of recovery would be expected to follow restoration of flow up to as much as 24 hours following the injury. Even if reconstruction is technically unsuccessful, collateral circulation may develop and be sufficient to nourish the bowel. Thus Ledgerwood and Lucas[11] report the case of a 19-year-old heroin addict who underwent resection of 2 cm of the SMA following a gunshot wound of the upper abdomen. This was followed by a prolonged period of mucosal necrosis and consequent malabsorption, but eventually there was good recovery. Aortography carried out at 10 weeks and at 2 years following the injury showed complete occlusion of the SMA with hypertrophy of the colonic circulation. The patient was found to be well at a follow-up examination 39 months after the original injury. There have been two other reports in the literature of prolonged survival following traumatic thrombosis of the SMA[3, 9] and, bearing in mind the astonishing capacity of the visceral circulation to develop collateral, it would seem probable that this injury occurs much more frequently than is generally suspected.

Arteriovenous fistula

There appear to be three varieties of this condition.

1. *Spontaneous* arteriovenous fistulae occur between the superior mesenteric artery and portal vein, in the region of the porta hepatis. This condition was first recorded by Goodhart,[6] whose patient was a 49-year-old woman with a history of abdominal pain and melaena. She was found at

Table 9.1 Mesenteric arteriovenous fistula following bowel resection

Reference	Sex and age of patient	Original operation	Interval	Symptoms	Course
Movitz & Finne, 1960[11]	F/34	Resection of strangulated bowel	4 months	Pain and bruit	Resection of fistula. Recovery
Munnell et al., 1960[15]	F/35	Resection for Crohn's disease	10 months	Obstruction; palpable thrill	Resection of a-v fistula + recurrent Crohn's disease. Recovery
Grafe & Steinberg, 1961[7]	F/67	Resection of obstructed bowel	6 weeks	Pain and bruit	Resection of fistula. Recovery
Durham et al., 1962[2]	F/37	13 operations for obstruction, followed by right hemicolectomy	3 months	'Buzzing' in abdomen	Resection of fistula. Recovery
Metzger et al., 1972[13]	M/24	Resection of strangulated bowel	15 days	Melaena	Resection of fistula. Recovery
Paloyan et al., 1974[16]	F/41	Hysterectomy, followed by volvulus and resection	18 months	Pain and bruit	Resection of fistula. Recovery

autopsy to have a fistulous communication between the splenic vessels, which had resulted in gross venous congestion of the colon. This was certainly the first case recorded of venous lesion of the colon leading to hypoxic damage. There have been several other cases reported since[13, 20, 21, 22] and the whole subject was reviewed by Stone *et al.*[20] who collected 38 examples from the literature, some of them spontaneous and some of traumatic origin.

2. *Gunshot wounds* of the abdomen occasionally lead to arteriovenous communications of the mesenteric vessels, which usually pass unnoticed at the time of the emergency operation, but become manifest later either because of intestinal symptoms or because of bleeding varices or because of the chance observation of an abdominal bruit.[17, 18]

3. *Iatrogenic* fistulae occasionally follow intestinal resection, particularly if mass ligatures have been applied to the vessels at the root of the mesentery. They may be symptomless or may cause epigastric pain, melaena or an uncomfortable 'buzzing' sensation in the abdomen.[2, 13, 14, 15, 16] Repair of the fistula, with or without additional resection of bowel, is usually straightforward (see Table 9.1).

Aneurysms

Nearly two-thirds of all splanchnic arterial aneurysms occur in the splenic artery,[19] and usually present as catastrophic abdominal haemorrhage. Provided that the patient can be brought in time to the operating theatre, splenectomy with excision of the aneurysm is usually a straightforward matter. Whether excision should be advised for the asymptomatic splenic aneurysm which presents as a calcified shadow on a plain abdominal x-ray, is more doubtful, except in the case of young women (especially in pregnancy) where operation is essential.

Aneurysms of the coeliac axis[4] and superior mesenteric artery are comparatively rare. Thus Stanley *et al.*,[19] who reviewed the literature in 1970, found only 9 cases of coeliac axis aneurysm (including 2 of their own), and 89 cases of superior mesenteric aneurysm (including 2 of their own). The authors advise an aggressive surgical approach to these lesions, particularly when they occur in association with bacterial endocarditis. They also draw attention to the occurrence of small, previously asymptomatic, aneurysms of the jejunal and colic vessels, which may present as acute abdominal haemorrhage ('abdominal apoplexy').

There have been a number of cases of successful excision of complicated visceral aneurysms,[3, 9, 10, 12] including the remarkable report by Haimovici *et al.*[8] of an aortic reconstruction which involved reimplantation of the left gastric, hepatic, splenic, right and left renal and inferior mesenteric arteries.

The detailed techniques of surgical reconstruction of these aneurysms are beyond the scope of this work, and will not be discussed further. The point should be made that dilatation of the coeliac and superior mesenteric arteries is very often a manifestation of widespread degenerative arterial disease, and the patient's fate and prognosis will then usually be determined by factors other than those operating in the visceral circulation.

External compression

Just as the coeliac axis may be compressed by fibres of the median arcuate ligament of the diaphragm, so the occurrence of fibrous bands which narrow the ostium of the superior mesenteric artery has also been reported.[5] It is doubtful whether such structures have any physiological or surgical significance.

References

1   Bole, P. F., Purdy, R. T., Munda, R. T., Moallem, S., Devanesan, J. and Clauss, R. H. (1976). Civilian arterial injuries. *Annals of Surgery* **183**: 13–23.
2   Durham, M. W., Robnett, A. J., Harper, H. P. and Yekel, R. (1962). Arteriovenous fistula of the mesenteric vessels. *Western Journal of Surgery* **70**: 9–10.
3   Fry, W. J. (1969). In: *Collateral Circulation in Clinical Surgery*, pp. 508–509. Ed. by D. E. Strandness. Philadelphia, Pa., and London, W. B. Saunders Co.
4   Garland, E. A. (1954). Aneurysm of the celiac artery. *Journal of the International College of Surgeons* **21**: 67–71.
5   Gautier, R., Barrié, J. and Sarrazin, R. (1965). Les angors abdominaux non-athéromateux. *Lyon Chirurgical* **61**: 893–894.
6   Goodhart, J. F. (1889). Arteriovenous aneurysm of splenic vessels with thrombosis of mesenteric veins and acute colitis. *Transactions of the Pathological Society of London* **40**: 67–70.
7   Grafe, W. R. and Steinberg, I. (1961). Superior mesenteric arteriovenous fistula following small bowel resection. *Gastroenterology* **51**: 231–235.
8   Haimovici, H., Steinman, C., Bosniak, M. and Spiegler, E. (1964). Excision of a saccular aneurysm. *Annals of Surgery* **159**: 368–374.
9   Kleitsch, W. P., Connors, E. K. and O'Neill, T. J. (1957). Surgical operations on the superior mesenteric artery. *Archives of Surgery* **75**: 752–755.
10 Kraft, W. O. and Fry, W. J. (1963). Aneurysms of the celiac artery. *Surgery, Gynecology and Obstetrics* **117**: 563–566.
11 Ledgerwood, A. and Lucas, C. E. (1974). Survival following proximal superior mesenteric artery occlusion from trauma. *Journal of Trauma* **14**: 622–625.
12 McClelland, R. N. and Duke, J. H. (1966). Successful resection of an idiopathic aneurysm of the superior mesenteric artery. *Annals of Surgery* **164**: 167–170.
13 Metzger, D. G., Hamilton, R. F. and Stephenson, D. V. (1972). Mesenteric arteriovenous fistula. *American Journal of Surgery* **124**: 767–769.
14 Movitz, D. and Finne, B. (1960). Postoperative arteriovenous aneurysm in the mesentery after small bowel resection. *Journal of the American Medical Association* **173**: 42–44.
15 Munnell, E. R., Mota, C. R. and Thompson, W. B. (1960). Iatrogenic arteriovenous fistula: report of a case involving the superior mesenteric artery. *American Surgeon* **26**: 738–743.
16 Paloyan, D., Collins, P. A. and Washburn, F. P. (1974). Superior mesenteric arteriovenous fistula. *American Surgeon* **40**: 481–484.

17 Rabhan, N. B., Guillebeau, J. G. and Brackney, E. L. (1962). Arteriovenous fistula of the superior mesenteric vessels after a gunshot wound. *New England Journal of Medicine* **266**: 603–605.

18 Spellman, M. S., Manda, L., Freeman, H. P. and Massumi, R. A. (1967). Successful repair of an arteriovenous fistula between the superior mesenteric vessels secondary to a gunshot wound. *Annals of Surgery* **165**: 458–463.

19 Stanley, J. C., Thompson, N. W. and Fry, W. J. (1970). Splanchnic artery aneurysms. *Archives of Surgery* **701**: 689–697.

20 Stone, H. H., Jordan, W. D., Acker, J. D. and Martin, J. D. (1965). Portal arteriovenous fistula: review and case report. *American Journal of Surgery* **109**: 191–196.

21 Sumner, R. G., Kistler, P. C., Barry, W. F. and McIntosh, H. D. (1973). Recognition and surgical repair of superior mesenteric arteriovenous fistula. *Circulation* **27**: 943–950.

22 Wheeler, H. B. and Warren, R. (1957). Duodenal varices due to portal hypertension from arteriovenous aneurysm—report of a case. *Annals of Surgery* **146**: 229–238.

10

Summary and conclusions

The experimental evidence shows that low blood flow in the intestine, whether this arises from local causes or from a diminished cardiac output, leads to physiological disturbances which at first are subtle and hard to detect, but later become gross and unmanageable. Almost certainly, this must have a clinical parallel. However, in terms of day-to-day experience, cases of manifest intestinal ischaemia are rare, and the average doctor may not see such a patient during his professional lifetime. Some would say that the condition is common but unrecognized, but this is to beg the question. Such special pleading has in the past been advanced for many 'diseases' which are no longer acknowledged to have a firm basis in pathology.

Quite apart from its being rare, mesenteric vascular disease predominantly affects the elderly, and it must be asked whether in a world whose main medical problems derive from malnutrition and overpopulation it is justifiable to devote any attention at all to such a condition. In other words, was this book worth writing?

In a recent symposium on the subject I put this question to three leading surgeons with particular interest in mesenteric arterial disease, and here are their replies.

G. W. Taylor (London): 'Although mesenteric vascular disease is rare, it does not always affect the elderly; a significant number of our patients have been women in their middle 40s with well localized aortic disease. I certainly think this syndrome should be kept in mind in any patient with otherwise unexplained postprandial abdominal pain, nutritional disturbance, weight loss, and abdominal arterial bruit.'

R. Kieny (Strasbourg): 'The question is essentially philosophical, and one needs to be precise about what constitutes an "elderly person". I would agree that intestinal ischaemia is quite often encountered in patients in their 40s. Furthermore, the bad reputation that treatment of lesions of the mesenteric artery has acquired is by no means justified. Early operation, before infarction has occurred, can have very satisfactory results. For instance, we reported 1 operative death in 35 reconstructions, and several 10-year survivals. Of the rest, 4 patients died within 3 years of operation, and 7 later. Causes of death were myocardial infarction (4 patients), cerebrovascular accident (5 patients), and renal failure (1 patient). Considering that the patients for the most part suffered from widespread degenerative vascular disease, these figures are not too bad.'

D. E. Szilagyi (Detroit): 'Offhand, I do not see the connection between the therapeutic problems of my elderly patients and the regrettable problems of malnutrition in many countries in which the rich eat too much and the poor eat too little, or in which the available meager public funds go into the building of atomic weapons rather than into sensible programs of public assistance for the hungry poor. Moreover, I do not see the relevance of being elderly and sick to the question of overpopulation. Obviously, the elderly do not contribute to the population explosion. Your question would be relevant if ischemic gut disease affected mostly, or only, the reproductive young. Then, if one were worried about overpopulation, one might let the young with ischemic bowel disease die. One might—but I would not. Overpopulation will not be corrected by euthanasia.'

For my own part, I cannot pretend to be unbiased, but I none the less feel that continued interest in the area of mesenteric vascular insufficiency is justified, both for the reasons given above and also because laboratory and clinical research into the problems of this very large compartment of the circulation must in the long term have an impact on clinical thinking. At present, the gap between physiologist and clinician is very broad, and it is one that only the clinician can bridge.

Acute intestinal failure

Acute intestinal failure is a condition whose causation, let alone treatment, we do not understand, although the development of the concept of countercurrent exchange in the villus has helped to clarify the situation. Once the mucosal defences have been breached and bacteria are invading the bowel wall, a chain of events is set up which it seems almost impossible to reverse. Recovery in established intestinal failure is at present virtually unknown, but this does not mean that the situation need be quite hopeless. There must surely be patients in whom the process is initiated and then resolves spontaneously without being diagnosed, and others whose lives are saved by supportive treatment given for different clinical indications. What is needed is on the one hand a high index of suspicion for early cases (and a method of identifying them) and on the other a realization of the measures we can take to prevent the process starting. At the same time it is probable that there is an irreducible mortality rate, in that necrosis of the alimentary tract is often rather a mode of dying than a cause of death, and represents the end-stage of multi-system failure.

Chronic intestinal ischaemia

The problem of chronic intestinal ischaemia, due to surgically correctable lesions of the major arteries, has preoccupied vascular surgeons and gastroenterologists ever since arteriography became possible. Over the years, however, the impression which has been borne in upon most of us who have been working in this field is that the patient whose abdominal pain is demonstrably due to arterial disease is exceedingly hard to identify. The criteria must be strict. It is not enough to observe a stenosis on an arteriogram, to reconstruct it surgically, and to accept thanks from the patient. The history of surgery is littered with operations which have been judged on such uncontrolled grounds and are now deservedly forgotten.

For the surgical procedure to be proved successful, it is necessary for there to be a quantifiable abnormality which correlates with the symptoms and which, following the operation, is shown to be abolished while at the same time the symptoms are relieved. Very few reported operations for supposed chronic intestinal arterial disease have met these criteria. This applies with particular force to the concept of the coeliac axis compression syndrome. However, as Dunphy originally suggested and as Kieny has subsequently shown, intestinal infarction is almost always preceded by a warning period, during which an elective arterial reconstruction should be life-saving. The technique of the reconstruction is important, which is why it was discussed in detail in the text. But how to select the patient with this type of disease remains our great problem, particularly as the resting intestinal blood flow will almost certainly be normal. It may even be that, before surgeons have devised an answer, their efforts will have been rendered obsolete by discoveries in the biochemical control of atheroma, so that chronic arterial obstruction to the gut, as in other parts of the body, will no longer require operation.

Focal intestinal ischaemia

Of less interest to the vascular purist, but of great significance to the gastroenterologist and general clinician, are the peripheral effects of focal intestinal ischaemia, whether in the small bowel or in the colon. The concepts of ischaemic enteritis and colitis have become firmly established, and are important not only because they differ in causation and behaviour from the granulomatous diseases, but also because they are curable. We now, for instance, know a great deal about the natural history and management of ischaemic colitis, and have learned how rarely is it necessary to operate in this condition. But is the whole idea wrong? Is what we clinically recognize and categorize as ischaemic colitis in fact anything to do with deficient blood flow? The pathological appearances are reminiscent of infarction, but it is unjust to the pathologist to expect him to define the cause of a newly documented disease process with his microscope, in the absence of hard clinical data. After all, we do not know what (except under very abnormal conditions) the blood flow in millilitres per minute to the normal human colon should be, and still less are we able to document low flow during an attack of ischaemic colitis. The major blood vessels are often seen to be open on angiography. These questions need to be asked, and are valid. None the less, there is a very strong body of circumstantial evidence both from the laboratory and from clinical experience that the changes in the gut wall are consistent with oxygen lack, whether mediated through large vessel occlusion or at microcirculatory level. Until another such hypothesis is put forward which fits the facts better than does the present one, it is pragmatically useful to regard patients with these now familiar syndromes as suffering from intestinal infarction. This implies a conservative approach to treatment, as regards both drugs and operations, and, indeed, when viewed and managed in this way, most of these patients get better.

The number of international conferences, invited symposia, research projects and published papers devoted to the subject of intestinal ischaemia has probably exaggerated its importance. None the less, the facts remain that vascular accidents do occur in the alimentary tract, and that they are potentially lethal and certainly underdiagnosed. The purpose of this book has been an attempt to put the subject in perspective.

Reference

Marston, A., Kieny, R. Szilagyi, D. E. and Taylor, G. W. (1976). Intestinal ischemia—a panel by correspondence. *Archives of Surgery* III: 107–112.

Index